The Ultimate (
Anxiety and

THE

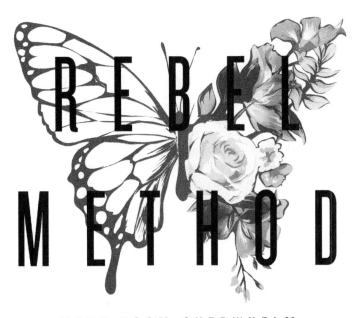

REBEL
METHOD

MOVE FROM OVERWHELM
TO PEACE OF MIND

Vanessa Wallace

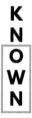

WWW.GET-KNOWN.CO.UK

CONTENTS

THIS BOOK IS FOR

Women of maturity and experience who have been high achievers and highly driven in their employment, but who have been affected at some point by someone close to them facing mental health or addiction challenges. They now want to take better care of themselves by finding freedom from the burdens, stresses and negative thoughts of everyday life before they are struck by the same problems. However, they feel lost as to how to move forward.

Those I work with and am writing this book for often feel resentful, unheard, overwhelmed, anxious, worried and in what they may call a dark hole or a dead end.

They probably don't really want to get out of bed in the morning, as it is just the same old, same old. They may feel they have lost faith in humanity after being let down.

They feel like they expected life to be sorted at this point and are disappointed it is not. They have a sense of 'why has this happened to me?'

A good day would be one with peace of mind and even a little bit of happiness.

- Do you want to take better care of yourself but find it is just not happening?

- Do you feel anxious or depressed?

- Do you find yourself ruminating on so many negative thoughts but you just cannot get them out of your head?

- Have you lost belief in yourself?

- Do you struggle to cope when challenges arise?

- Do you wish you could put yourself first for once in your life but don't quite know how?

- Do you feel you can't carry on like this and are ready to give yourself a chance to be happy?

Do any of these questions resonate with you? If they do, then this book can certainly help.

I have worked with over 100 amazing women who have come to me answering yes to at least some of these questions. As we worked together, I guided each of them through a process to get to living a life of their dreams— whether that meant being free of stress and negative thoughts so they could live with hope and peace of mind, or improving the relationships in their lives to feel they had a true purpose– and I am excited to take you on that same journey in this book.

To get us started on our time together, why not try this little questionnaire? It will only take you a couple of minutes and it will help you to find out which parts of my REBEL method will be the best for you to have in your life. Of course, all of it could be helpful, but different life relationship types will find different parts of the REBEL method more in line with their needs at any given time.

All you have to do is point your phone's camera at this QR code below. It will then open up a link for you to sign up for all the resources linked to this book.

THIS BOOK WILL

Open doors for you to the possibility of a better life, with freedom, peace of mind and loss of that sense of 'if only' or 'I should have done better'.

This book will take you from a place of negativity and overwhelm to one of hope and serenity. Calm.

- You will find yourself able to wake up with some peace of mind in the morning.

- You will be able to control that 'monkey brain' – or 'washing machine brain', as I sometimes call it. The one that keeps going over and over things but just does not come up with any solutions.

- You will be able to place your head on the pillow at night feeling confident that you have been OK that day, as much as possible.

- You will be able to accept the things that have happened to you in the past.

- You will know that every day is a new day, and you have the chance and opportunity to make it better.

You are not a bad person, you never have been, but the voices tell you that you are. It is not true. Some days you get an inkling of the fact that you are better than you think, but it is so faint. This book will help you to build that voice that tells you that you are OK, because you are OK; like everyone else, you have your flaws, but they are in no way worse than other people's flaws. Your brain has just got stuck like a broken record, and it is not your fault.

In this book I am going to take you through a series of steps based on my REBEL method. This method will enable you to:

- **R**emove that inner critic.

- **E**ducate yourself about what is really going on with your mind and brain so you can understand and not be so harsh on yourself about it.

- **B**e yourself now. Stop always putting others' needs first and neglecting your own; be confident in yourself and who you are, and learn to put the past behind you.

- **E**liminate anxiety and depression. Allowing yourself to be you, and following through on that, will make you feel so much happier. Anxiety and depression will begin to slip away as you implement all the tools in this book.

- **L**ive the life you dream of. This is not about fancy holidays, huge amounts of money in the bank or the dream home and partner; it is about being content with yourself, having peace of mind and quieting the negative thoughts in your head so you can just have a break!

MEET VANESSA

So who am I? I have certainly had quite a chequered past and struggled myself with anxiety, depression and addictions. I have also been, in the past, a chronic pleaser of others, full of low self-worth and without any self-belief. Sometimes I would not even speak for fear of being 'wrong'. Now I am a workaholic, a mum to three wonderful young people, a grandma to two beautiful granddaughters, and the owner of a black cat and two pugs. I got married in 2010 to a wonderful man who completely accepts me for who I am.

I now live in rural Northamptonshire, which I love. My favourite thing about it is the canals. When I was a child, we used to go for trips on the canals. They are so peaceful: the calm water, the ducks, moorhens and swans, the odd kingfisher and the sound of the boats chugging along. I used to love how that sound changed when you went under bridges or tunnels, how the sound used to echo off the walls. I would often stand under them and shout, listening to my voice bouncing off the bricks. I was able to hear myself, something I was really quite afraid of most of the time, but it felt exhilarating in those moments. Perhaps those walls would hear me...

My parents are both dead now. My father was a consultant surgeon, my mother a nurse. She worked on the front line on the wards in London when the soldiers came in from D-Day, and would often speak of that experience. My dad was posted to Scotland during the war, and it was always a family joke how he got off so lightly, basically living in a household where he was heartily fed lots of Scottish porridge and really saw nothing of the war.

My father was very encouraging for my brothers and me to study hard in life. I do thank him for that now, but at the time it made me a bit resentful that I had to come back to university at the age of 19 when I was having a whale of a time selling boxer shorts on the beach in Lanzarote. That was my first business enterprise!

Anyhow, I scraped through my initial studies in psychology and anthropology with a third-class degree and, by that point, a chronic amphetamine addiction. I was miserable, living in squats in London, but thought I was cool and living the life I wanted. In fact, I was just rebelling (hence the REBEL method) against conformity and responsibility; I just wanted to be in a fantasy world all the time. I did not like this real life – it all felt too difficult.

Cutting a long story short, after reaching rock bottom in 1999, resulting in a period in rehab, there followed a journey of recovery and realisation, self-awareness and self-development, until I became a therapist in 2005. There will be more on that in a later chapter. This qualification led to me working in prisons, rehabs and for homeless charities.

There were three points in my life when I made significant shifts in who I am as a person. Funnily enough, all of these were 10 years apart. Number one was after a bad car accident in 1998, when I spent lots of time laid up recovering from some quite serious injuries. During this time I enrolled on a counselling course. It was a revelation; I realised that I had choices in my life, something I had not understood before. Suddenly, I knew I could change my life if I wanted to. At the time I was feeling pretty hopeless, negative and overwhelmed with my life. In fact, I had got to a point where I did not want to go on living any more; even though I did not have the courage to take my own life, I felt so stuck. The counselling course gave me some insight into the fact that I could change my life path if I wanted.

The second one was in 2008, when I was ill for a period with swine flu. I was in a high-pressure job which involved working many hours. Life at home was not easy. I was constantly stressed and quite depressed. I had started taking some herbal remedies to manage my depression but was waking up feeling so dark and bleak every morning. I was thinking, 'is this it? Is this what my life has become?' Even though I was away from the chaos of addiction, my life was not right. I felt dissatisfied, incomplete, like I was living a life that other people felt I 'should' live, and I did not like myself. I was constantly anxious about sharing my voice and truth and felt I was just swerving from one crisis to the next.

During this time, I started to look at some coaching tools. I came across a really cool exercise that looked at each area of my life and asked me to score how I was doing in them. There were quite a few where I scored really low. I realised this was why I was so unhappy, so I made it my mission to start to develop myself personally and be more in alignment with who I really was. This was not an easy journey, but piece by piece– learning new things, getting new help, going back into counselling and coaching– I started to feel so much better.

You could also try this exercise. The diagram below shows areas in life. Score each one on a scale of 1 to 10, 1 being an area to improve and 10 being an area that is fully fulfilled. This will allow you to gauge the areas that you need to build on and get help with. You can also access this exercise in the pdf document on the resources page, which is accessed via the QR code below:

Your Life Satisfaction

Imagine the cups below are areas of your life.
Think about how satisfied you are with each area, and colour in the cup accordingly.
For example:
If you are 100% satisfied – fill the cup!
If you are 50% satisfied – half fill the cup
And all percentages in between!

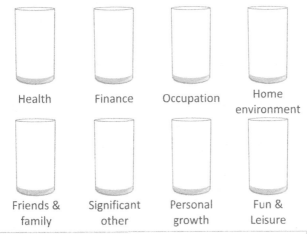

Health	Finance	Occupation	Home environment

Friends & family	Significant other	Personal growth	Fun & Leisure

What changes I can make to fill some of those cups I would like to be fuller:

My most recent transformation was in 2018 when I was launching my business, having been let go by a company I was working for. It's a long story but was definitely an example of there being a silver lining to something which seemed quite catastrophic at the time. In fact, if that had not happened, I would not be here writing this book today.

During this period, I learnt about crystals, colour therapy, meditation, yoga, feng shui and energy healing. These areas enhanced and reignited my belief in the spiritual side of life. I started to meditate and journal every day and practise yoga – and I wrote this programme, the REBEL method. The REBEL method is in complete alignment with what I believe and have experienced to help with our mental health. It provides freedom from the darkness of depression and anxiety.

I gained a coaching qualification and stepped into my own power, doing what I truly wanted to do with my life. I started to run retreats based on the REBEL method, and I have never looked back.

WHAT PEOPLE SAY ABOUT ME

'For anybody that hasn't been on one of Vanessa's retreats, I've been on one just under a year ago now. I was very reserved, I didn't know what to expect, but it was the best thing I've ever done. It's made me open up and make some peace with my thoughts. I would highly recommend it. It's amazing. And it's been a lifesaver for me. I was in a very dark place a year ago. And, you know, thanks to Vanessa, I am a different person now.'

– THERESA

'This experience was incredibly valuable and has really helped me to think about my feelings and ways in which I can help myself.'

– JANE

'I attended a retreat just over a year ago. It took me a couple of days to really open up but once I had, there was no stopping me. I've done quite a lot of work with Vanessa since then. I would highly recommend it. I found it very grounding, and it made me think about the things I do every day and why I do them. I've used the tools and techniques so many times since. Absolutely well worth it. It's very therapeutic and very cathartic. I would highly recommend it.'

– SARAH

'Enlightening! Many light-bulb moments for me. I came to realise and more deeply understand why I react the way I do. This in turn helps me find the path to change for the better. It was also good to be with people who similarly struggle; sharing their experiences was lovely, offering a real sense of there being a safe space in the group.'

– HELEN

'I arrived at the retreat not knowing what to expect. On the outside I had the perfect life – family, friends, home, career. However, on the inside the hate, negativity and criticism I had for myself was all-consuming, dominating everything I thought and did. Each of the workshops led by Vanessa, Lorna and JJ were enlightening, exploring why, allowing us the safe space to self-reflect, and offering techniques and opening awareness to change. It wasn't easy. It was deeply challenging, and for me very emotional. But there were so many light-bulb moments. There was continuous support at the retreat in the form of amazing people, a restful environment, delicious and nutritious food, a wonderful massage, and yoga as I have never experienced before. I have felt an overwhelming shift in myself already, and I look forward to the future. The previously negative thoughts were now replaced with positivity, mindfulness, acceptance and self-compassion, to name just a few. Thank you.'

– SHARON

If you would like to learn more about our retreats, please do feel free to visit my website:

www.crystalclearcoaching.org

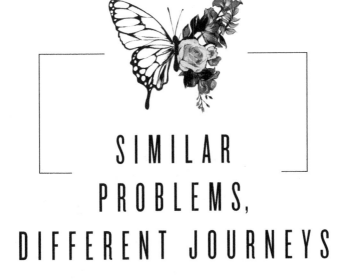

SIMILAR PROBLEMS, DIFFERENT JOURNEYS

"Be of good cheer. Do not think of today's failures, but of the success that may come tomorrow. You have set yourselves a difficult task, but you will succeed if you persevere; and you will find a joy in overcoming obstacles. Remember, no effort that we make to attain something beautiful is ever lost."

– HELEN KELLER

M eet Theresa.

Theresa was flustered and hot as she arrived at my retreat. After a difficult and anxious journey to get to us, during which she nearly turned back and went home, she arrived at the retreat centre and literally fell through the door, shaking, emotional and in pieces.

She had got lost on her way to us, but somehow she had found the drive and energy to push through and keep going. She knew she needed help and that things desperately needed to change following a turn of events in her life. If she did not take that step, she could not see herself still being around in a year's time, as she said to me. It had all become too much for her; living on a daily basis had become excruciatingly painful.

We gave Theresa a cup of tea. She sat down on one of the large sofas in a heap, a look of complete exhaustion on her face. The whole effort of the drive had left her depleted of any resources. Her face looked pale, anxiety was written through the tightness in her brow, and her eyes were devoid of any spark. This woman needed caring for, someone to nurture her back to safety and instil some hope. She needed someone to tell her that everything was going to be OK, because she had lost all sight of this notion.

This lady had a story to tell. She was a successful schoolteacher who felt that it was important to not bring any personal issues into work. In fact, she prided herself on her professionalism. Theresa saw vulnerability as a weakness and was always careful to make sure people thought well of her. The thought of people not liking her or viewing her as not doing a good, even perfect, job crippled her with anxiety.

The issue was that, ever since Theresa was a child, she had been given the role of carer. As an adult, this extended to her husband and children, the students she taught at school and her parents. When her husband got diagnosed with a bad stroke, it felt like the last straw. She felt she had never in life had the opportunity to do anything for herself. She felt quite resentful about this, and thoughts of caring responsibilities she had had as a child kept popping into her head, fuelling this feeling.

Theresa had been through some massive life changes recently, including some health problems of her own. She was desperate to have a good life but felt so set back by her husband's illness. Her depression and anxiety took serious hold, and she also was experiencing powerful and overwhelming urges to run away from it all.

Since her husband's diagnosis, she struggled to see a way forward and had found herself slipping into negative and obsessive thinking. She felt like her life had come to an end and that everything was completely hopeless.

She was finding herself avoiding going home as much as possible to avoid dealing with the situation there, which she was finding overwhelmingly difficult. She joined a gym and ended up just sitting in the car park or the café for hours just to avoid going home. She did not really know what she was avoiding but had this strong urge to just run away; her deepest desire was to have no responsibilities any more, as she felt she could not cope. She felt so guilty about these feelings and thoughts she was having.

Every day felt like a struggle, and the panic and anxiety attacks were getting worse. Sometimes she just found herself in a heap in tears on the floor when people weren't around to see her in this state.

Theresa knew she needed to talk about things and how she was feeling but did not want to burden her friends and colleagues and was unsure whether she could trust them. She was also discovering that they were often not helpful and did not say what she felt she needed to hear. She felt that she was letting everyone down.

Theresa fluctuated between feelings of anger and guilt. These two feelings were tightly intertwined: often the angry feelings led to guilt for feeling angry and then back to anger at the situation she was in in her life. The anger resulted from her having to do everything for everyone else and the guilt for feeling resentful about that.

Theresa is not alone with her problems. I come across people so often who are struggling with similar issues, such as guilt, anger, wanting to escape, anxiety and depression.

There were a few key problems for Theresa:

1. She had taken on the role of carer throughout her life, so looking after herself was not familiar to her.

2. She had a belief that she needed to be strong.

3. She was worried about what people thought of her.

4. She had just been through a massive trauma with the sudden change in the health of a family member.

5. She had previously struggled with depression and anxiety.

6. She was currently overwhelmed with very negative feelings.

7. She felt hopeless about her life.

Theresa is not the only one to have come to me with similar types of problems. Time and time again I see older women who have successfully ploughed through life being highly professional and supportive of others who suddenly crash, sometimes because of what seems like a minor problem (though, of course, in Theresa's case it was not so minor). However, sometimes our previously maintained ability to function and get through life's difficulties just breaks, and it is actually nobody's fault. It is similar to a sponge that has reached saturation point: our bodies and minds suddenly decide they cannot take any more.

Of course, the cost to anyone who reaches this point is catastrophic. It can lead to an inability to function in one's career. People in this state often lose out on time with family members, elderly parents, grandchildren or grown-up children.

Another consequence is the loss of dreams and plans. When surviving the present takes all your energy, there is none left over for dreams and plans. Most of us think that as we get older, we will have more freedom and financial stability, and therefore more time to spend with family– but when we are tortured with negative thoughts and feelings, this does not seem so attractive and actually can feel impossible to maintain. Our expectations of how life should be at a later age are destroyed, leaving us feeling deflated that our life has not turned out how it could or should have.

This has not come about through any weakness or failure on your part, or even on Theresa's part. Like a sponge, you have absorbed so much over the years that now you are at saturation point. The brain does not take kindly to an overworked life. In earlier times we would have been in the minority if we lived beyond the age of 45. In 1900 both men's and women's average life expectancies were between 45 and 50!

So think of all the extra years of brain functioning and work we add to a lifetime these days; for most of us at 45–50 years of age, our careers peak, as do the pressures. But just over 100 years ago, we would not even have expected to be alive at this time.

Are our brains really able to take on these extra years without a break? I think not.

Many people who come to me (and perhaps you can identify with this yourself) have not had simple lives. Perhaps childhood may have been a little difficult, marriages were problematic, or perhaps they had to care for others throughout their lives, placing an extra strain. Perhaps their career had proved to be particularly challenging, or they had to manage addictions in their family of origin (their parents) or in a partner or a child, or even addictions of their own. All of these situations put a strain on a person. Sometimes my clients have felt that their lives have been ruled by someone highly dominant and controlling; this in itself leads to really negative feelings and high levels of two hormones: cortisol and adrenaline.

So let me talk about these two hormones.

Essentially, when we deal with difficult situations in life we produce hormones in our body in response to our feelings. You may have heard of the 'fight or flight' response. This is when you are on alert, adrenaline is produced and you are ready to deal with a situation that may appear threatening (e.g., failing). The fight or flight response helps you to perform better, so it is quite useful too, but when you are in it all the time it is dangerous and not good for your body and mind at all. Cortisol levels start to build.

Cortisol enhances your brain's use of glucose and also curbs functions that would be non-essential or even harmful in a 'fight or flight' situation. In response to this hormone the fight or flight response shuts down other areas in the body (e.g., digestion, rational thinking). This can cause headaches, depletes the immune system and basically stops all normal functioning while you deal with the threat. Your heart rate goes up, you may sweat a lot and your breathing becomes laboured or very fast.

So lots of things are happening to our body when we're in the stress response. The problem is that when we are in the fight or flight response for most of our lives, we are constantly producing hormones in our body that are needed to help us deal with situations but also cause damage to our bodies and minds.

In the short term, your concentration and focus will be affected, and you may have stomach problems or headaches. In the long term, constant secretion of these hormones into your bloodstream leads to anxiety and depression, concentration problems and sleep problems. Even if you do not experience anxiety and depression, the concentration problems and sleep problems can lead to you feeling that you have less control in your life, which in turn can lead to depressive feelings and an underlying anxiety.

Now, if you have either a person or a situation in your life that is difficult for you, we could blame that situation or person. It is true that this is a strain on you; you are the one producing these stress hormones, and you are the one left feeling so overwhelmed. However, blaming that person or situation only makes your anger worse, which then triggers more stress hormones.

The same happens if you blame yourself. This is also very stressful on the body and mind. Recognising the situations in your life and how they are impacting you without blaming yourself is key. It is not your fault. Your body and mind are in overload from this stressful situation.

Previous traumas or difficult times in your life, which most of us have had, can also affect your brain's ability to cope, and can resurface at any time, even though you may feel you have dealt with them. You may have pushed a previous trauma or difficult time to the back of your mind and felt like you have dealt with it well, but the brain has the nasty habit of remembering these traumatic events when anything slightly similar occurs in later life. Also, a previous trauma can have a profound effect on your whole body and your mind's coping mechanisms.

The reason you are feeling the way you are is a combination of factors outside of you – your life circumstances and situations (either in the past or present) that have affected you – and your internal chemistry and the ways in which your brain processes information and stress.

With all those external and internal factors, it really is no surprise that someone like Theresa would be suffering.

The good news is that this problem is solvable.

I have been taking people through my REBEL method, from the start to the end point, for over 10 years now. I have worked with people from many countries and with many different occupations and life stories, but I have got them all to a place where they have a peace of mind and an ability to manage and understand their difficulties. I am so passionate about helping people like you. This is because I know it is possible to get through these times and come out the other side. I am living evidence of that, and so are many of my clients.

It would give me such joy to know that you, too, were able to come out of your dark place and find some peace so you could then go on and live a happier life, engaging with your family and finding activities that you enjoy as well as being at peace with yourself. It is my duty now to show this to people, as it is a process that can literally save lives.

It is OK to struggle, but you are not alone. Many people have struggled in a similar way to you. You can do this; you just need a helping hand and, having picked up this book, you are already on that journey to getting the true you back, with me holding your hand along the way.

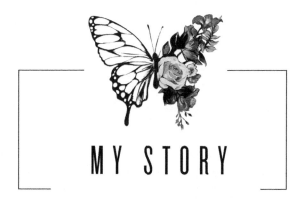

MY STORY

*"Only in the darkness can you
see the stars."*

– MARTIN LUTHER KING

I t was 28 March 1998, in the middle of the afternoon. I woke up in the car, people around me. I looked down to my right; the side pocket of the car door was full of blood. I had been involved in a bad car accident. It turned out that a drunk driver had come over onto my side of the road and hit me head on.

The weirdest thing about this was that the night before, I had said a prayer – something I don't do very often, because

I am not really a believer. Anyway, the prayer (or cry for help) was a combination of 'I can't live like this any more', 'get me out of this' and 'I just want to die'.

I had been maintaining a heroin addiction for three and a half years. Struggling to cope, I was desperately addicted to a substance that I could not stop using, trying to bring up three kids in the midst of it and trying to make ends meet. During this time, I had made frequent attempts to stop with trips down to stay with my parents to detox myself– which were followed by a return to life with the children's father, who was also a heroin addict. I would always end up caving in and using drugs myself again, almost as a means of self-medication to deal with the pressures. I was trapped in a situation where I could not get clean and stay clean.

Life was miserable and dark, and all the time I was just squashing my potential, my spark, my passions and my ambitions. I really could not even contemplate achieving anything, because in my mind, I was unworthy. After all, I was just a junkie! I felt so horrible and ashamed of myself and my life but, to deal with these feelings, I would just use more drugs.

Back then, 24 years ago, I did not know how things could change. I felt there was no hope for me. I believed my kids would grow up and I would be a sad old lady, stuck at home with no career, no prospects and no money, rejected by society for being such a failure. I saw myself as hopeless, totally unable to fulfil any of my hopes and dreams for my life. I had resigned myself to my inability to move forward in my life at all; this was how it was going to be, and there was no way out.

I could not control my mood swings and would dip into despair at the slightest of triggers, or even with no trigger at all – I would just suddenly feel awful, angry, frustrated and highly emotionally unstable, sometimes getting urges to just kill other people or myself (I was not capable of this, by the way). The words 'I hate my life' would often come out of my mouth.

I always had this gnawing sense, though, that there was something better for me in life.

WHERE IT BEGAN: CHILDHOOD

I did not just arrive at this point in my life suddenly. I had been brought up in what would seem a 'normal' family. There was a good amount of money around; my father had just qualified as a consultant surgeon around the time I was born, and I was the youngest by quite a few years. My father was a cancer surgeon and saved many lives. He was always focused on prolonging and providing quality of life and went over and above for his patients.

At nine years of age I went to boarding school. I might have ended up in the same position in later life without it, but I do believe that it played a big part in me developing an ability to 'shut down' my emotions, get on with it, be the good girl, and not cause any bother.

Boarding school was full of routine; there was really no time for nurture or conversation with those who were supposedly caring for us. It was either music practice, meal-time queues, lessons or after-school study in the dining room, with some allocated television time later in the evening. Then bath times, bedtimes and lights out at scheduled times. The routine was tiresome and laborious; the same thing every day, no variation and no one to talk to. There was no parental support, just rules and regime. Bells rang for every occasion, and strict timings were in place for every activity: mealtimes, music practice times and even times when we were allowed to eat sweets.

I started to keep secrets about how I felt– but there was no one to tell them to anyway, and so it was easier to just shove all feelings down. After all, you had to get on with it.

By the age of 14 I was smoking cannabis down at the bottom of the school field. This was fun! I was going away on my 'exeat', as they were called– weekends when we were supposedly allowed home or, in reality, to the houses of other students' older siblings, where there were parties and drugs and wild times. This felt good at the time, offering a time out from the pressure and frustration of being the 'good girl'. I just needed a release from all of my time playing the perfect daughter, friend and student to keep everyone happy.

So the rebel in me came out!

Essentially, I wanted to run away from anything that 'conformed'. I had an attitude of 'I will show them!' My father had always called me 'Little Miss I'll Do It' in my childhood, and I think this came out loud and strong when I was a teenager. I suppose I felt abandoned in some way and decided I would take control of myself and do things my way because I saw no benefit in what I had experienced so far with the strict routine and suffocating control of the boarding school environment.

So the rollercoaster started: drugs and parties and squats and travel. I was having a whale of a time, or so I thought. What had started as a fairly harmless teenage rebellion grew into a full-blown drug dependency in four years.

TRYING TO CHANGE: EARLY 20s

During this period I always had been interested in psychology and, after gaining three A levels at school despite being a nightmare to my parents and constantly being out at night and partying, I lived for a year in the Canary Islands. There were lots of parties, but then I returned to England to attend university to study anthropology and psychology.

Time at uni was still an ongoing party, and I am not proud to say that during this time of living in squats and attending lectures erratically, I met the father of my children and became pregnant quite quickly with my eldest son. I completed uni, scraping through, and was awarded a degree eventually after a year out to have my baby. I then joined the travelling community in Wales, attending festivals, taking drugs, living in vans and buses.

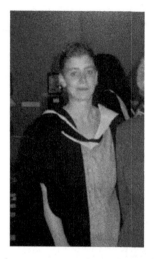

1991, graduating from university with a 3rd class degree in Anthropology and Psychology and a severe amphetamine addiction.

By the time I was 25, I had three kids and was living in a cottage in Wales; my drug use had become habitual and eventually led to dependency. It wasn't about the teenage parties any more; it was now about coping on a daily basis and self-medicating my feelings so I could be stable – or what I thought was stable. I was working as a chambermaid and also doing some bar work, but it was all pretty tough, as I tried to juggle these things with a chronic heroin addiction at the same time.

I had responsibilities that I wanted to meet but just could not. I was addicted to drugs and needed them to function on a daily basis, so they became the most important thing, the priority. I was failing not only myself but everyone around me: my children, my parents and other people in my family.

I felt so desperately fed up with the lifestyle, the daily need to find drugs just to feel normal and the constant arguments, the lies to my family, the depressed feelings, the negative and suicidal thoughts. There was disappointment on my children's faces every time I was late to pick them up from school because I had been out trying to score drugs. I just did not want to live any more if my life was going to be this way. I thought my life was just hopeless and I often imagined myself just wasting away as an old lady drinking brandy and sipping methadone to keep me on an even keel and to numb the pain.

This was when the car accident happened. Essentially, it was my wake-up call.

There was a gift that came to me at this point as I lay on the hospital bed with two broken arms, bruised legs and a massive head injury. It was an awareness, a realisation that I did not want to die and that actually I was slowly killing myself with the drugs.

But I needed help and, at that point, I found the courage and humility to ask for it. I got off my 'I'll do it' pedestal and decided that I could not do it alone. I admitted to a few people that I was struggling, and I started to get some help.

I was placed on a methadone programme and, while laid up in bed convalescing from the accident, I started searching for something – something to get me out of this desperation and depression I had found myself in. I wanted to learn about myself, and so I started to read about counselling. Having already completed a degree in psychology, it made sense for me to carry this on. I signed up for a counselling foundation course.

I can quite honestly say that something had shifted within me following the accident and I wanted to seriously change. I had an excitement in my belly as I started to see that there might be hope and a way out.

One of the first things I had to do was get out of the relationship I was in, because my partner was an addict. It was not doing either of us any good, and I was certainly not going to stop using drugs if I stayed with him.

I must admit this was one of the hardest things I have done, other than coming off the drugs. We were extremely wrapped up with one another, and I had also become his carer. To illustrate my feelings for him, here is a diary entry I made about our relationship in 1989, almost 10 years before the accident that changed everything: 'James has brought some beautiful things along in life for me, we have beautiful times together and we have a beautiful son.'

This entry was followed by the chorus lyrics from the Rolling Stones song 'You Can't Always Get What You Want'.

I was deeply in love with him, but the relationship had been full of turmoil as a result of our addictions and the constant drug use. The lies and manipulation that go on alongside addiction were destroying us both as individuals and causing so many problems, fights and arguments in the relationship.

By this point he had been admitted into hospital with chronic pneumonia as a result of his drug use, and I was being asked by the staff at the hospital to have him back home to care for him. To leave him in such a bad way was extremely difficult, but I had to do it for the sake of the kids and myself. I needed to get well.

It was a dark and rainy winter day when I walked away from the hospital, never to return to the relationship. My heart was so heavy, but I knew it was the right thing to do for both myself and the children. With the help of a family member who gave me some words of encouragement to walk away, I turned my back on him and never went back. This was a highly emotional point in my life; it was tough to do. I did love him, but I needed to live, and I knew we were both going to die if I stayed. He eventually died, in 2016, from the impact of addiction on his body.

I got myself a place in a drug treatment centre after several failed attempts to come off the drugs on my own. The whole family had to move, which was a massive wrench for my children at the time; they had to go and live with other members of my family while I went into treatment. They were distraught and deeply affected by the move.

Treatment was not easy. It was challenging. I had to learn about myself, my behaviours, my emotions and my thinking, which was chaotic and irrational as a result of my lifestyle, attitude and drug use. However, the programme was successful, despite a couple of small relapses. I ended up in a very good women's 12-step treatment centre in

North London, and my journey to freedom from addiction was given such a boost there. In fact, I owe my life to this place; I never used drugs or alcohol again after entering that treatment centre.

TURNING THINGS AROUND: REALISING I COULD CHANGE

When I got back home after being in treatment for nearly a year, things were not easy – but I had the support I needed and the tools that I had learnt in treatment.

My self-esteem was low. I constantly doubted myself and I had so many feelings about being a bad parent as the reality of the impact of my addiction on my children started to come to light. However, all I could do was move forward, so I got some voluntary work and tried my best to do right by my children and everyone else around me. There was a lot of anger around. I was angry, my kids were angry, my family were angry, and we all had to pick up the pieces and move forward.

I felt vulnerable, fearful of my future and unsure whether I could make it. I worried all the time about what people thought of me. I lacked boundaries and was always saying yes when I really should be saying no. I still felt worthless and undeserving, perhaps even more so than before, as I now did not have the drugs to medicate this feeling.

Following this, though, there was a period of getting it together for me. I realised I was struggling with a lot of anxiety and depression and my drug use had been about medicating this, so without the drugs I was left with these feelings. I spent the next five years getting counselling. I joined groups and made friends with people I could talk to honestly about how I felt, because they had felt the same and they understood. It was such a relief to me, finally being able to speak frankly about my emotions.

I started to see some light and hope for my life. It was a slow process, and sometimes I would take ten steps forward and eight back, but I was getting there. I felt inspired and motivated to learn more about myself, my feelings, my thoughts. The more I learnt about myself, the more I wanted to learn, and the better I felt. I had a strong hunger to experience how I could live a better life and feel better on a daily basis. I was like a sponge, soaking up all the new tools and ways to cope with feelings, thoughts and my own destructive behaviours. It was not an easy time – in fact, it was really challenging; there were lots of tears and frustrations. Eventually, though, I started to feel brighter within myself, like a weight was gradually being lifted.

My incessant desire to learn, understand and gain clarity on what I was going through led me to read up about rational emotive behaviour therapy (REBT). This was the most logical approach I had ever come across in managing my stress and anxiety. I had always loved science at school, and this approach was so scientific and so logical and easy to implement into my life. I explored it more and found that it provided me with a formula to stop beating myself up and accept myself despite my past, and also to manage my intense feelings on a daily basis. As someone who loved maths, the clarity of having a formula for change and managing emotions was so attractive to me.

In fact, I enrolled on a master's degree in this very subject.

FINDING A PURPOSE: PRISON

During this degree we were asked to find a placement somewhere so that we could gain the client contact hours necessary for working as a rational emotive behaviour therapist. I started at a women's centre but had also been looking into prison work. I felt drawn to this. I think just the knowledge that either myself or my ex, or both, could have ended up in prison for the things we did to support our drug use made me want to help other people who were in those circumstances. They could not particularly control some of the elements of their lives, but they ended up with massive consequences from them.

I met a lady on the master's who was currently working in a prison, and she introduced me to a voluntary organisation that provided counselling for prisoners. After an interview, I was accepted as part of the team. I was so excited and nervous at the same time, but absolutely thrilled, too; for once in my life, some of my dreams were coming true.

It was actually terrifying. For the first few months, I was so anxious going into the prison. I was scared of doing the wrong thing, of messing up, of letting someone out by mistake or not remembering to lock a door, but I kept going in – and every time I worked with a client, I got such a great sense of satisfaction.

Eventually, I secured a role on a six-month residential therapy treatment programme for addictions within the prison. This was an intensive service; we ran group therapies every day. The success rates of the organisation I worked for were very high.

It was intense work, draining and rewarding at the same time. A community of its own. A place where people got well. We shared tears, celebrations, disappointments, anger, frustrations and disciplinaries. I can quite honestly say it was the most rewarding role I have been in for any charity or organisation. I learnt so much about running groups and managing the dynamics within them. I learnt to understand people on a deeper level, how to be really compassionate and understanding and to just be with people in their distress and not judge or criticise. I must admit that I have many of these qualities anyway; I have always been able to connect with people empathically and feel compassion. However, this took me to a different level of being able to be alongside people who are really in distress.

Sometimes I could come away with a deep sense of satisfaction because I had helped someone in some way: given them some hope, provided them with a space to let their emotions out, given them some realisation, or organised the session where they had that moment of clarity,

45

that time where it became absolutely clear how they could move forward in their lives. In addition to that, I loved the days when people left prison with a new sense of hope; I would meet them again at the head office where they were volunteering, getting on with their lives and being back together with their families.

Apart from working in the prisons, I worked for various rehabilitation centres for addiction and charities. During that time of running workshops, gaining experience and training, and trying different methods with clients, I developed my formula, which I feel is the quickest and most effective route to turning your life around and feeling better on a daily basis.

I started working with others, showing them this approach, and I saw results. I knew addiction was simply a coping mechanism that many had developed to manage emotional difficulties and numb their pain. Having the opportunity to teach others how to cure their emotional difficulties was such a pleasure. I loved seeing clients' eyes light up as they got that moment of clarity and realisation, understanding that they could change how they were feeling about circumstances in their lives. I could see people becoming happy again. It was such a wonderful feeling to ask the question at the beginning of a session 'How has your week been?' and to hear for the first time, 'Actually, I have had a really good week this week. I have been OK.'

I recognised that self-acceptance was central to a person's recovery, as it had been to mine. I started to study self-acceptance on a deeper level and even wrote a thesis on it for my master's dissertation.

In this part of my journey, I was so excited. Of course, I was nervous at the same time, but I was absolutely thrilled that, for once in my life, some of my dreams were coming true. In the years after my residential treatment, there were good days and bad days, but even in the dark days I knew it was worth it and I was getting closer to the life I wanted. I was moving towards the purpose of my life.

THE FINAL BREAKTHROUGH: CRYSTAL CLEAR

In early 2017 I was working as a manager in a rehabilitation centre for addictions when they suddenly 'let go' of me. I was distraught, shocked, rejected and extremely disorientated. What was I going to do now? For the first time since I had started working properly in 2005, I was without a job.

My resilience was strong, so I was able to turn this around quite quickly once the tears had stopped and the anger subsided. Within a couple of weeks, using the tools that I had learnt and have now shown to so many other people, I was able to change my problem into an opportunity. I started to think 'right, what can I do now?' I had been thinking about setting up my own business for many years but just did not have the confidence; I had always believed it was something for other people, not something I could do. I also had a belief that I needed a degree in business studies to have my own business. That was what my father had always told me, and I believed him. A boss at one point also told me you needed to be a certain type of person to run your own business. I was not sure exactly what he meant, but I did understand that he was telling me I was not that type of person. However, I had few other choices at this point, so I decided to write a programme and, with my passion and belief in residential settings as great places for recovery, Crystal Clear Coaching and Retreats and the REBEL method were born.

Crystal Clear Coaching and Retreats, using the REBEL method, were set up to help people move from overwhelm and fear to peace of mind and hope for a better future. It is the most life-changing programme I know of. It works! It helps you to feel better, live better, have better relationships and be able to function with happiness, confidence and peace of mind. It helps you to manage emotions and negative thoughts. It addresses the past and provides for the future. It tackles that inner voice— the one that can tell us we are no good and can destroy everything and any prospects. This is the REBEL method!

Setting up on my own was something that was actually unimaginable from where I had come from. I had previously been the addict who was just hanging on and doing bits of shift work here and there. But something within me, my intuitive self, told me I was doing the right thing. I had such passion and belief in the programme. It took me all of a week to write. I knew the exact formula I would use, as I was living proof that my methods worked and I had seen countless results in short periods of time for other people.

Now I work with women and men who have perhaps 'functioned on the outside' throughout their whole lives, even though they are working in important jobs, perhaps even in senior management roles. These clients of mine know that underneath the competent exterior, they are dealing with some issues that have not been resolved. Consequently, there have been points in their lives where they 'crashed', feeling unable to cope, but somehow they have managed to pick themselves up and carry on. Now that has stopped working for them, and all the walls have tumbled down. Life seems dark and difficult; all hope has been lost, and that previous belief of 'I can do this' has changed to 'I really can't do this'. With that comes another feeling: 'What is the point of being here if I am unable to function and sort this out?'

I know how it feels to be in this dark place.

I support my clients to pick themselves up from that dark pit. I give them the hand that they need. I walk with them along the way and gently and compassionately do for them what they can no longer do for themselves.

We work together to understand the problem and to piece together a sense of hope. I show them how to manage their feelings and thoughts so that they can function... and also how to start to really put themselves first, perhaps for the first time in their lives.

I discovered through my work what makes a difference, what are the essential tools we need, and what shifts we need to make to get well and live a happier life. From this I developed my formula, the REBEL method. I absolutely believe– and my experience has proven me right– that this is the most effective route to turning your life around and feeling better on a daily basis.

ANNIE'S STORY

Annie came to me for help in 2020. Her husband had become very ill with a complex neurological condition and his whole personality had changed. Things had become so difficult for her. She felt powerless. She had a sense of loss, a real lack of control in her life, and the walls had come tumbling down on her seemingly perfect life.

Annie had been a highly functioning person throughout her life: a mum, a teacher and a wife. She had always prided herself on her problem-solving abilities and, even though life had inevitably had its challenges, she had always been able to move forward and deal with problems with an extremely practical focus, usually devoid of emotion but with the goal of supporting everyone to move forward. She was always determined, and smart in appearance, priding herself on her very professional look and attire. She had a beautiful family, wonderful grown-up children, and grandchildren she doted on. There had been a plan for retirement – enjoyment, travel, less pressure and more time with family – but then the accident happened.

When Annie came to me, she was distraught, overwhelmed, hopeless and feeling like her life was over. She felt she had no one to turn to and had lost trust or hope that any help would be coming her way. Physically, emotionally and spiritually, she was completely broken.

As we got into the sessions, she identified periods in her life when she had felt despair but had been able to brush it off, piece herself together and move on. But now she was unable to function; she was in despair, questioning her whole existence and purpose. She had always been able to think herself out of problems, but this was different. Her feelings were overwhelming. She was wondering what life could be like going forward and feeling that all was lost. She wanted help and, for the first time in her life, she asked for it.

After working with me for a few weeks, Annie was able to calm down the overwhelm and find a space to reflect on her life. She made some big decisions, placed boundaries and started to see a way forward. She was out of her dark pit and now saw a life ahead with hope.

We will read more about Annie's story and how she found renewed hope in Chapter 6.

YOUR STORY

I am writing this book because, if you are like Annie, I would like you to know that you too can move from overwhelm into hope, you can manage your negative thoughts and feelings, you can come out of that dark pit– but you need help to do it. I can compassionately guide you, accept you for who you are, not judge you or tell you that you are a failure. I can help you to understand why you feel the way you do and hence to see a path out of your dark place. I can help you to find hope within yourself. The time clients spend with me is not easy, but they report that it is honestly the best thing they have done for themselves.

'If you think you are not ready for this kind of thing, you really are… It has changed me totally.'

– SARAH

'I feel so much lighter, more positive and better equipped to deal with whatever life has in store for me. Would highly recommend Vanessa to anyone looking for a helping hand in getting them through a difficult time.'

– KEELEY

Knowing that people can come out of that hopelessness, and being able to show them how to do that and see the results, is the most joyful and rewarding experience for me. I feel it is a gift that I have been given and it is my duty to give this to as many people as I can in what is left of my life. Hence my company has been born after years of preparation, and more and more people are seeing a way forward, getting the transformation they deserve.

If you identify with any of the feelings and issues I have described, or with Annie, you absolutely deserve this too. You do not have to struggle; that is not what life is here for. If you are looking forward and feeling hopeless, I know that feeling and I also know that you *can* get over this hurdle. It may be the most difficult thing you have ever done in your life, but I absolutely believe in you.

Like my father, I believe in the idea that everyone deserves a better quality of life. My father dealt with physical ailments, while I work with the brain but, in a way, we are so similar. If there is something wrong physically, then we go to the doctor and get help. Our brains can also become broken, but with modern science and understanding, we now know there is a way to heal the mind. I have had the privilege of being able to do this for myself and now have the even greater privilege of showing others how they can do it too.

My programme incorporating the REBEL method takes about three months. It includes online workshops, face-to-face three-day retreats and one-to-one sessions as well as self-study courses. With these elements, I take people through each of the steps. Once my clients get to the L of the REBEL method, they have hope of a better future, one in which they will be living the life of their dreams.

Check out my website **www.crystalclearcoaching.org** for more information.

GETTING READY TO REBEL

'Yesterday I was clever so I wanted to change the world. Today I am wise so I am changing myself' – Rumi

Prepare yourself for a journey towards being a true mental-health rebel (in a mindful way, of course).

Are you ready?

How do you know you are ready?

Are you sick and tired enough of being sick and tired?

Do you have a motivator?

Perhaps you look at that person next door and see them happy, or perhaps you look at other people whose lives are seemingly OK and who seem to just 'float' through life? This makes you envious initially… but then, hey, there's a wake-up call! *You* can do something about it. Perhaps you have just reached a point in your life where you cannot go on any more as you are?

It is not going to be easy, so this is why I ask you: are you truly ready?

Are you ready to feel like s*** some days but still push through? Are you ready to accept compliments from others? Are you ready to push aside self-doubt and that nasty voice on your shoulder saying 'you don't deserve this'? (Of course you do!) Are you ready to push aside that voice that says your old ways were better?

Perhaps you have thought about the legacy you want to leave behind?

Do you want to be seen as someone who overcame adversity? Do you want to be like Victor Frankl, who survived a concentration camp, or Nelson Mandela, who was imprisoned for years but still found a positive mindset? This may seem impossible, but your legacy can be a good motivator. Think about it; how do you want to be remembered by your family, friends and those who loved you— perhaps even by those who did not love you?

On the note of family, perhaps you have children you want to do this for? You want to set an example, and you want to change the script in your family in regard to how you all deal with poor mental health or dysfunction.

On the other hand, you may want to do this because you simply want to feel better and feel that you cannot go on any more feeling the way you do.

All of this might seem quite challenging, but we do need a good reason to change because, essentially, the brain resists change at all times. This book can help you.

Throughout the book you might hear me talking to your brain as if it is another person. I have always found this a useful way to explain things. After all, our brains are like computers: they churn out what we give them. Your brain is resistant to change because not changing things is comfortable and 'safe'.

To help you with this and to help you override your resistance, which *will* come up (it is only natural and everybody has it), try doing the exercise 'cost/benefit analysis' in the pdf that accompanies this book.

Follow the QR code below to get your free resources and book pdf:

I do this 'costs of change' analysis with many of my clients. We get a sheet of paper, divide it into four parts and put these questions in the four boxes:

- What are the benefits of your position now?

- What are the costs of your position?

- What are the benefits of change?

- What are the costs of change?

Download the pdf and do this exercise yourself.

Here are some of the things that people come up with for the costs of change: sadness, fear, having to be vulnerable, struggle, pain, boredom, loss of family/ friends, anger, having to face the unknown, not being in control... the list goes on. What are your costs of change? There will be some. This means you are completely normal, as we all resist these types of changes. It may seem ridiculous that you are resistant to changes that may benefit you, but this is just the brain trying to do its job. By doing the exercise and pushing forward with this, even though it may feel hard and like you are walking through treacle, you will be teaching your brain that this type of change is good, especially as you start to get the positive results.

You need to do this preparation work, because some days you are going to want to give up. But rebels disregard the 'norm' and do something different, so I know you will keep going. On the harder days it will seem like your old ways were easier: going to bed for the day, avoiding social contact, not going out of the house, not speaking to anyone, not exercising, eating crap food or denying your feelings. All of this will seem more attractive to you at times. But you need to remember your long-term goals.

Just a note here on the inner critic, who we will be talking about later on in this book. Now, the inner critic may jump all over a bad day and tell you how badly you are doing, that you are not worthy of feeling better, or what a failure you are for even thinking of not taking care of your mental health for a day. *Ignore* that inner critic. It is telling you lies. Your inner critic teams up with that part of your brain that tells you change is a dangerous thing. But if you have a bad day or two or three, it's OK. You have made progress already by getting this far and even by reading this book.

WHAT YOU WILL NEED

It will be useful for you to get a few things before beginning your rebel's journey of mental health recovery.

Get a notebook and write down how you are feeling in the morning, afternoon and evening. Becoming aware of your feelings is key; you can use the feelings chart in the book pdf to help you with this.

Start to write down the things that you appreciate in your life (e.g., sunshine, Diet Coke, chocolate, your partner, your home, your garden, flowers, nature, a pet… literally anything that you appreciate). Keep it simple. This is all you need to do for now.

Other useful items, although you do not have to get these yet, are:

- A puppy – not essential for all; for some it may be a garden, a few plants or even some colouring books or crafting kits

- Someone to help you declutter your home

- Good healthy food

- Someone who knows what you are doing and that you intend to work on your mental health.

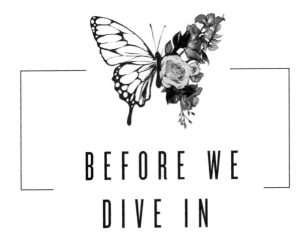

BEFORE WE DIVE IN

When people make enquiries with me and I ask them what help they have had before, they tend to fall into two categories.

The first type of person is someone who has been for counselling before, perhaps even for many years, but has found that it is not helping them move forward. They may say it was useful because talking about things has helped them feel better and the counsellor tends to listen to them and reflect back how they are feeling, which gives some comfort, but it does not help them move forward out of the situation they are in. This type of counselling is called person-centred counselling and certainly has its place; I have used it myself when I was struggling with three teenagers at home. I felt I had a place to offload my frustration and have a good cry.

However, many people who come to me and have had this type of counselling feel it has not been what they really needed. They say, 'Surely there must be more I can do?' My answer to them is, 'Absolutely, yes – there is. There are tools and strategies you can learn beyond just talking about your problem.'

The other type of person I talk to is the client who has been for cognitive behaviour therapy (CBT), often via their doctor. They will say one of two things:

1. 'Yes, it was great. I learnt the tools and they were really useful, but then I forgot about them when my problems came back.'

2. 'I was just not in the right place to take on board the techniques at the time, so I didn't get much from it.' (This person was clearly overwhelmed and just unable to concentrate to the level required for CBT techniques.)

These problems have occurred because CBT on its own is great, but more is needed. You need to address what is going on across so many other levels. The REBEL method helps you to do this.

You may be wondering if the REBEL method will work for you.

Perhaps you just think it is too difficult to do; you have tried other methods and nothing has seemed to work. It has become so energy draining going into therapy so much.

The REBEL method deals with the blocks first. This makes it so much easier and more effective. You cannot keep walking down a path if you have gale-force winds trying to push you back all the time. These gale-force winds are resistance. We all have it. Resistance to change is such a common thing to have and it is so normal. It is a natural human thing, but once we tackle it, you will find yourself sailing through the rest of the steps. You can start to feel a lot better quite quickly, which will consequently help you push on with the rest of the method. You can feel like I did when I was hungry for change, enjoying my recovery and life again.

Let's address some of the most common questions people ask me when they are unsure whether the REBEL method is for them.

WHY IS IT GOING TO TAKE ME SO MUCH TIME (WHICH I HAVEN'T GOT)?

How much time do you need to live a better life? You have a choice here: continue as you are and spend the rest of your time feeling the way you do, or invest some time to rediscover your quality of life, living your time happier and with peace of mind. You will be amazed by how, once you start on this journey and start using the tools, your life can change so quickly. As long as you do the homework, you can gain some really rapid results.

WHAT IS THE COST?

Yes, it will cost money – but again, this is an investment in your life, your quality of life. We can all buy a better bed so we can sleep more comfortably. Likewise, we can buy a better washing machine so our clothes are nice and clean, making us feel fresh on the outside, but what about investing in feeling better on the inside every day? We do need help with this – it is not generally something that just goes away. The financial investment provides you with quality of life, happiness with your friends and family, resolution of relationships, employability, clear thinking, and hence the ability to develop your career. There are so many returns on the investment.

AM I BEYOND HELP?

No, you are not. You have just not tried this approach before. The problem is that when we try lots of things and then they don't work, we get the 'I am different' syndrome. And you are absolutely right: we are all different. That is why an individual approach is needed, as happens with the

REBEL method. However, you are not so different that you are beyond help. If you apply the methods and work at them with the help and support you will receive here, then you will feel happier, more balanced and calmer.

The brain always comes up with rationalisations as to why we shouldn't change. It is just trying to protect you. But this is the one time where you need to tell your brain something different. After all, the evidence is there: hundreds of people have recovered with this method, and so can you.

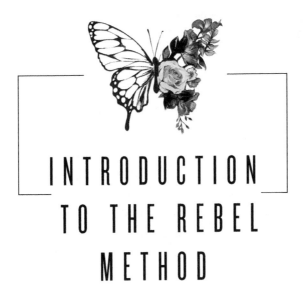

INTRODUCTION TO THE REBEL METHOD

"If you do not know where the leak is, you cannot fix the plumbing."

– VANESSA WALLACE

WHAT IS THE REBEL METHOD?

The REBEL method is a clear roadmap to help you move from overwhelm to peace of mind.

It supports you on your way. It is simple and involves science, techniques that work and a way to live your life that supports you so much that overwhelm becomes a momentary, occasional blip in your life rather than a crippling chain or wall that stagnates your progress and impacts your life negatively.

The REBEL method is not just for rebels; it can be for ordinary people who have found that life has just got too difficult and they want change now! That's the rebel in you – you have had enough of being sick and tired.

It is a process, and following it involves learning tools and reusing them at times so that you can keep moving forward. Once you know the elements, they will come to you as easily as learning to ride a bike, and you will be able to quickly implement them to get you back on track if you feel a slip coming on. That is why the method is so effective: it is simple, and there are some real basics that, if you do them every day, will cause your life to change and get better.

The REBEL method is the template I use with all my clients, whether I'm working one on one, in a group, at a retreat or even online. The template evolves through the work we do together because, while working with me, my clients will address all areas of the REBEL method.

When I first went through the elements of the method with one of my clients, Katherine, she said, 'Oh my gosh, that is me! That is exactly what I have had to do.'

The REBEL method is what I use in my life. I totally live and breathe it myself. It has been my journey from overwhelm to peace of mind. In the past, I was the most negative (and hence overwhelmed) person you could ever meet. I needed all of the components of the REBEL method.

The first three parts (the R, the E and the B) are action steps. The final E and the L are what you get as a result of doing R, E and B, with some added tasks and tools along the way. When E and L start to not be present in your life any more, you go back to R, E and B and look at what you are missing out on, or what you are not practising in the REB steps. It's as simple as that.

Sounds easy, huh? It *is* pretty easy… once you understand it.

HOW DID IT COME ABOUT?

I have been developing my REBEL method since getting into my first unhealthy relationship and becoming addicted to drugs in my twenties. I was dissatisfied with my life but could not work out why.

I was in a desperate place back then and experienced so many negative feelings. Here is a quote from my diary on 30 November 1988: 'How can I even start to explain how I feel at the moment? I feel like someone has placed a lump of cement in my stomach.'

I quite often had moments where I felt like this. With hindsight, I believe they were the result of depression and anxiety, but I did not see it as that then. I was only 20 years old. I was always an academic, a deep thinker, someone who liked to work things out logically, but I could not work out why I felt so bad all the time. There was nothing particularly difficult about my life.

I needed to get myself better but had to learn a few key skills to do that. The techniques I learnt to feel better, move forward, get out of the overwhelm and live a happier life are all now components of the REBEL method.

These included placing boundaries in my life, both with other people and with myself. I also had to have some compassion and start being kinder to myself. I needed to ask for help and accept help. All of these things I had shied away from before. Understanding how my brain worked, and knowing what I could do to rewire it, was the key; all of this was absolutely life-changing and has been life-changing, too, for my clients.

In the early years of my recovery, I went on to work in prisons with offenders who were stuck in cycles in their lives they really did not want to be in any more. I watched and saw how some found a way out. I observed how they spoke in the groups, and the tools they used. I then saw which ones started to really make progress in their lives – the ones who went on to become positive and productive members of society. I worked with some of those people as they then became volunteers and workers for charities, giving back to others what they had learnt.

I was inspired by their stories and wrote a thesis on the key areas I saw as being fundamental for change in my clients. One of these was self-acceptance and finding a way to quieten the destructive, negative internal criticism and self-talk. I was so excited by my findings and found clear evidence of my theories being right; there was a direct link between building self-acceptance – removing the inner critic – and recovery.

After years of working in prisons and institutions, I lost my job as a manager of a rehab, and it felt as though things were just in sequence and ready for me to progress into making this unique and transformational programme for people who were really struggling, just as I had done in the past. My coaching training was due to start. My understanding of cognitive behaviour therapy was combined with my learnings about how our mindset and attitude towards ourselves can be such a factor.

At this point in my life, I had to put my own tools into practice. I had to get out of my own way, looking at how my beliefs about myself were holding me back. I went away on a business coaching retreat with my coach, Carl Brooks, and learnt about stepping into my own power, allowing me to be myself. The feeling of authenticity and empowerment

I gained from this was amazing. I became so passionate about giving others this opportunity to step into who they really are and who they are truly meant to be. I have mentored many people over the years, watched them grow, letting go of what was holding them back, and harnessing the confidence to embrace what inspires them, leaving behind their critical voice that tells them things must stay the same. Watching this evolve with people I have worked with has left me with such an unbelievable sense of joy.

One day, I asked for feedback from my peers, as instructed by my coach. What came back from the people I asked were the words that now stand on my email signature: 'powerful compassion and understanding'. Wow, wow, wow! This gave me such a sense of pride and belief in what I was doing, beyond any achievement in my life previously. I absolutely knew that I was here to help people find their happiness. Strangely, when I was a young teenager at a church service with a family member, a lady came up to me and said I had a purpose in life which would be shown to me. I suppose this may be what she meant – who knows?

It certainly does connect to my heart as I watch people recover, the smiles returning to their faces, the tension in their brows relaxing as over time they let go of the stress. I feel so grateful for this gift of all the years I have been able to spend training the hundreds of people I have worked with, and also the gift of my own recovery journey providing me with the template for the REBEL method.

WHY THE REBEL METHOD?

So what is so special about the REBEL method – or, in fact, even the idea that it comes from me?

First and foremost, it aims to be deeply compassion-ate and understanding of you as a person. It is unique to you but drawn from a template that really works. It helps you to understand what is going on, why you feel the way you do. A lot of other methods take you straight to the solutions. I am not talking about taking you deep into your childhood here – that is just way too scary for most people – but simply understanding what is going on in your brain and why you are feeling the way you are. There is always an explanation, and it is so important to be compassionate and kind with yourself about that explanation, because beating yourself up for feeling this way is not going to make you feel better. In fact, it is only going to make you feel a lot worse.

The REBEL method gives you a level of clarity that gives you absolute permission and the ability to know what the next steps are. It gives you power: the power to move forward in your life.

HOW DO PEOPLE FEEL WHEN THEY WORK WITH ME?

I have had a few people who have said I saved their life.

Days get easier. Intense negativity starts to become less frequent, and positive experiences become possible.

You will find yourself starting to do more things and starting to enjoy them again.

You can start to feel free, empowered and educated. You will understand what is happening when you feel bad, so you will have the power to take control again because you will know what you need to do.

The REBEL method addresses the root cause, not just the symptoms. It knows the science behind why you are the way you are but also how the science and your personal life story and history have moulded together to bring you to where you are today. Once you understand this, you are then given clear methods to make the changes you want to make; whether that be to feel happier, have more motivation, reduce your negative thoughts, manage your emotions or reduce your feelings of overwhelm.

The REBEL method is different for everyone, because we are all different individuals, but it works for everyone. In a way it's just like clothes: we all need to wear them, but how we wear them or the colour they are can be different for everyone depending on our taste, personality, beliefs, how we feel on the day and where we are going or want to go.

The story of how the REBEL method came about involves one of those serendipitous moments we all sometimes have.

I was in conversation with my coach and we were building a new website for Crystal Clear Coaching. She asked me what were the key things that I do. I stated, 'Help people to remove the inner critic, be themselves and live the life they truly dream of.' And she said, 'We have an RBL method there!'

My mind got to work immediately on this. I love a play on words, so I said, 'Well, if we put two E's in, we have REBEL!'

I have always been a rebel myself; I rebelled in school, I rebelled against my parents, I rebelled against living a 'normal' life. Because of this, the word 'rebel' was really appealing to me.

The E's were easy to find. First, I strongly believe that education and awareness are key. Understanding how the brain works, knowing what is going on and why we feel the way we do or why we react or think the way we do has always been such an area of curiosity for me and was fundamental in my recovery journey (and those of others I work with).

Eradicating anxiety and depression is my end goal for all my clients. Now, let's be completely realistic about this. Completely eradicating it may be a long shot for you, but it's certainly true that finding a place where it is not impacting your life so much any more *is* achievable. Being able to live days when you feel great and not entombed under a wall of anxiety or depression, being free and having peace of mind, is absolutely possible, even if you think you are beyond repair.

So this is how the REBEL method came about. It is the ultimate toolkit to wellbeing, to living the life that you dream of every day, to having peace of mind, to being free of anxiety and depression.

WHY DOES IT WORK?

It focuses on removing blocks

The REBEL method works because it focuses on removing blocks. We can all go and read a self-help book with lots of tools to get better but, for some reason, we often find we still just can't move forward – or we make some progress, start some new habits but find ourselves slipping back into the old ways. This can often leave us banging our head against a brick wall, wondering why these things are not working for us and perhaps really beating ourselves up for our apparent failure.

However, this struggle is not your fault.

The reason you are struggling to maintain the new skills is that your blocks are holding you back. So again, I repeat: this is not your fault. Blocks are powerful and controlled by our brains, often despite ourselves.

This is why the REBEL method helps, because it starts by removing the blocks – the bit that so many other approaches do not do. Believe me, before I discovered the REBEL method and removed my blocks (the R and E part), I would continually try new things and find myself going back to my old ways, leaving me feeling even more frustrated and disappointed in myself.

So, it works because it removes the blocks first. It removes those areas that hold you back, those areas that keep you in a repetitive cycle. The ones that leave you in a position where you think you have changed... but find yourself six months later going back to your old ways, the negativity creeping back in again.

It helps you build self-compassion

The REBEL method supports you to understand your thoughts, emotions, beliefs and reactions so that you can be compassionate with yourself. Compassion is so key, and is actually the only thing that started my journey. As long as I was harsh on myself and condemned myself, which was within my family culture, I could not move forward. Negativity and self-criticism was my default mode.

Let me explain this in another context.

A lot of diets– and especially restricting ones– do not work, because the brain reacts to them as if they are a threat. If you limit your food, feel hungry all the time and eat food that you genuinely do not enjoy, eating becomes a negative experience. Your brain sends out warning signals, and the body consequently starts to store fat because it believes you are in a famine or a crisis and is reacting to that perceived situation. Essentially, your brain starts to act on its own to 'save you' from potential death.

It is the same if you approach change with negativity and criticism. I had a particular client, Claire, who had personally struggled with years of criticism from her parents, leaving this as the default mode in everything she did or didn't do. So, even when I started to work with her, she was still not moving forward. We discussed this in more depth, and it came to light that Claire was highly frustrated with herself, beating herself up on a daily basis that she was not moving forward quickly enough. This was a major block for her, and we had to overcome it before she was going to be able to move forward. She was getting in her own way with her negative self-talk. She needed to be compassionate with herself and much gentler, as she would be with someone else who was struggling. Once we had overcome this block, Claire started to come on tremendously and began to feel really proud of herself. She was also happy with her life as she started to make changes and put in boundaries with people who were destructive to her self-worth.

When we try to bring in new techniques for wellbeing, the brain does not like it. It does not like change; even if the change is something beneficial, it will revolt against it. Claire had been so used to being this way with herself, because it had been instilled in her from a very early age. Her body and mind were completely rejecting the idea of being compassionate with herself. However, that is exactly what she needed to do. We worked on various exercises to help her to do this.

Claire's situation was extreme: she actually felt sick and visibly squirmed at the thought of doing something nice for herself. As she had constantly been criticised throughout her life, she saw herself as undeserving of positivity; it was a completely alien thing to her; in fact, it felt so strange to her that her mind completely rejected it. Our brains see changes to our way of being as a threat and send out alarm messages. Claire was one of the most giving and kind people when it came to other people, but she needed to give some of that to herself. She understood this, but needed to work through the discomfort it was giving her, with my help. We started with small steps and built it up. Claire started to feel so much happier in her life within a matter of a few weeks.

The REBEL method helps you to understand your blocks and work with them, to be compassionate with yourself and not to beat yourself up. This is absolutely key. Progress will not happen while you are still being harsh with yourself.

WHO DOES THE REBEL METHOD WORK FOR?

Let me tell you about Kate. She came to my retreat two years ago, but we did have a few phone conversations beforehand.

I clearly remember where I was when I had my first telephone conversation with Kate. I was in the car, and the phone rang. I pulled over to answer it, thinking it was someone calling about an appointment I had set up for myself. But instead, a lady was on the other end of the phone in tears. She said she had seen my retreat online and needed to get away for some space for herself, because she was completely overwhelmed with life and under a lot of pressure looking after her mum, who was going through cancer treatment. Kate also told me about how she had lost her first husband to cancer a few years previously and had not felt supported during this time by anyone, but had to push through it as she had a young child to think about. Kate told me she was not coping. She was feeling over-whelmed all the time and was resentful that she had to help her mum, but also felt guilty if she didn't.

Kate had children to look after at home, a husband she felt unsupported by, and a high-pressure job. She was trying to maintain her home, look after the children, keep her job going and look after her mum and dad all at the same time.

Kate cried a lot. I just listened.

I listened intently to what she had to say on this call, and we agreed that she would have some telephone sessions with me. Video calls were not something she wanted to do; they would be too challenging, plus she did not like seeing herself on camera and said she would feel too exposed.

So how did the REBEL method work for her, and what were the steps and points in her journey of recovery?

Kate had a massive inner critic. In fact, it was the voice of her mother. This had been there for so many years that it was not easy to get rid of. Kate had to make her own voice stronger than that of her inner critic, but her feelings about herself were also really low. She desperately wanted to be listened to. She felt no one listened to her or even saw what she needed – it was like she was invisible. I helped Kate to become visible, to understand that her brain was under the influence of so much conditioning from others and from her childhood. She had been bullied at school, too, which did not help.

The expectations on Kate were overwhelming for her; she always pleased everybody, always wanting everyone else to be OK, so she was not used to thinking of herself, which meant it was hard for her. After all, her inner critic would tell her she was being selfish.

So we worked through all of this. Kate attended workshops on self-care and self-belief. She gradually started to be OK with being who she was. This was a sensitive person, perhaps quite different to a lot of the people around her in her life. She learnt to nurture that side of herself and take care of herself, and once she had realised what she needed, she started to put in boundaries with others. This was a big step!

Kate's anxiety and depression started to slip away. She had happy moments and peaceful moments. She started to sleep better and was no longer waking up in the night with negative thoughts and things going round and round in her head. She started being who she was, stating what and who she was to other people – especially at work – and found that it was not so bad doing that; actually, it felt empowering and good.

Kate's dreams when we first met were to just not be overwhelmed, to be able to function, to not feel unhappy all the time and to stop hurting herself. She achieved all of this and continues to work on maintaining being Kate and being OK with herself and her life as it is. She has been able to let go of past resentments and the pain of loss, and has begun to see her life ahead of her as a new adventure, moving into a new phase of freedom and time for her.

If you are overwhelmed, stressed, burnt out, anxious or depressed, the REBEL method will work for you.

If you have a dysfunctional family background or have had an incident in your life that has set you back, the REBEL method will work for you.

If you have a history of broken relationships or high expectations of yourself, the REBEL method will work for you.

THE REBEL METHOD: A BIRD'S-EYE VIEW OF THE JOURNEY

The R represents: removing the inner critic

The inner critic keeps us stuck. It is made up of negative thoughts that make us feel overwhelmed, and it needs to be put in its place. Just telling it to go away will not work, though. We need to build a relationship with it and understand its position. Now this may sound a little 'woo-woo' to you – having a conversation with your inner thoughts – but your inner thoughts wire your brain accordingly, a bit like a computer. So whatever you feed into your brain, it churns out. This is actually part of our survival system, but it gets in our way because it is just too loud sometimes, or we listen to it too much.

In this book I will show you how to manage your inner critic so that you can be less self-critical, feel better about yourself generally, allow yourself to receive compliments from others and start doing some nice things for yourself in among all the stress you are experiencing.

You may ask why you would want to do that; my answer is that by removing your inner critic, you will take away the thing that blocks you from moving forward. Removing the inner critic will help you to progress to peace of mind so much more easily, as you will be able to press forward and implement things in your life that are going to make you feel better without that negative voice of imposter syndrome holding you back. You will feel generally happier– and once we are happier, our motivation builds, so getting on with your day will feel like less of a chore. That wall of negativity will slip away, giving you the space to see life ahead and have hope for your future.

The E represents: educating your mind

This is vital. As I always say: if we don't know where the leak is, we can't fix the plumbing. It is the same with our brains. If we do not understand why we have these unhelpful reactions, thoughts and emotions, or where the leaks or miswirings are coming from, then we don't have a hope of fixing them. With this part of the method, I will educate you about your thoughts, your emotions and your behaviours. You will learn and understand why the way your brain works is not your fault and that on numerous occasions it operates automatically without your input. It responds to your environment, situations and experiences and produces a reaction.

I will teach you how to override these programmes in your brain, but this step will also give you the awareness to be able to name and identify what is going on in your mind, giving you more control and reassurance that you are not going crazy and that your mind is actually trying to do a job for you. I will show you how to teach your mind to do a job that serves you better and how to decipher between real and perceived dangers.

The B represents: being yourself

Imagine being truly yourself. How would that feel? You only have one life – why spend it pleasing everyone else?

Another thing related to the way our brains work is that we often are not authentic, because it can feel vulnerable or risky. But happiness comes from being ourselves. This is because when we are being ourselves, our stress is less and we can 'flow' more easily through life. Part of this is being able to accept ourselves for who we are, as well.

Not being yourself has so many negative consequences: people-pleasing, resentments, anger, lack of self-acceptance, or beating yourself up about your actions, behaviours, thoughts or emotions.

First of all, learning to be yourself may be a road of discovery, finding out who you really are, what you really like, what is authentic for you. This is an exciting journey.

I will support you to discover who you really are and what really matters to you in life. I will help you to develop strategies to become your true self and to cut out the areas where you are simply pleasing others, to your own detriment.

The E represents: eliminating anxiety and depression

I am not one of those gurus who believes they can instantly cure you of anxiety and depression, but I am a great believer in the fact that we can gain the tools to reduce and essentially eliminate any anxiety and depression on a daily basis.

Anxiety and depression come as the results of difficulties in life, overwhelming problems, unhelpful patterns from our past, and thinking patterns that can hold us back. I will show you a toolbox of strategies with which you can identify the root of why you feel the way you do, and then show you techniques that work to reduce your negative feelings and thoughts, leaving you able to function on a daily basis on a more effective level. We will look at your patterns, and perhaps explore the history of your life if you feel able and willing to do so. We will identify what does not serve you and help you to eliminate those things, with compassion and understanding and no judgement, of course. We have all had hard things happen, and acknowledging them is important.

This is the step that is individual to you, to your story. I build a relationship with you so I can understand who you are. I really listen to you. I am only concerned with who you truly are and what your hopes and dreams are, and I support you and guide you to see what holds you back. This might feel quite scary, but don't forget that at this point you will have already achieved the REB part of the model; this step is fine-tuning that and providing you with a foundation for recovery in the longer term. This step deals with the root and aids you to manage your anxiety and depression for the rest of your life.

The L represents: living the life you dream of

Do you just wish to wake up with peace of mind every day? Well, this programme will give you that.

Having gone through all of the steps, you will be able to really understand what you need, apply it in your life and be the person you are truly meant to be, as well as living a life filled with contentment and happiness.

Sounds like a pipe dream? Well, I am living proof that the REBEL method works. I was a hopeless heroin addict with no self-belief and so many blocks in my life. I was depressed, anxious and stressed. I felt hopeless. I believed I could never move forward. I was constantly getting in my own way. With the steps in the REBEL method, I now live the life of my dreams. I understand my brain, anxiety and depression, and I use the tools to enable me to keep going and to manage them on a daily basis. Not every day is wonderful – there are difficult days, but I know how to get through them now and can turn things around very quickly from a bad day to a good day. I am much more resilient and can 'ride the waves' of difficulties in life.

So are you ready for this journey?

There are no exceptions. If you are perhaps thinking that this will not work for you, how can you know that if you have not tried it? I believe in you and have great hope for you, especially since you have got this far in the book. I honour you now and completely support you on this journey. You have found a special place here. Your heart could be bursting with enthusiasm for life in the next few months.

WHY DO I FEEL LIKE THIS?

Because it is absolutely my mission to enable you to have a better quality of life. The idea of that just gives me so much joy, and it is also my life's purpose. Essentially, that is why I am here on this earth and have been through what I have been through – so that I can show *you* how to change your life.

CHAPTER 5

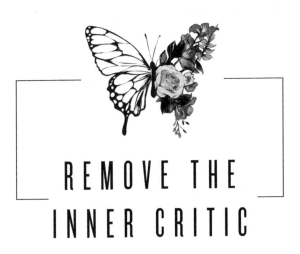

REMOVE THE INNER CRITIC

"You have been criticising yourself for years, and it hasn't worked. Try approving of yourself and see what happens."

– LOUISE HAY

My inner critic used to be so loud. I used to feel completely swamped with self-doubt and shame. My inner critic would stamp all over something I did or planned to do.

One Christmas really early on in my recovery, when I had just come out of a rehabilitation centre for drug and alcohol addiction, I was at the dinner table with my family. There were quite a few of them— my brothers and their wives, my parents, some nephews and nieces. I had at the time received much support from my family: helping me in the early stages of my recovery, looking after my children, being supportive of me and generally helping out. All of this was so I could concentrate on myself and my wellbeing while I was in rehab.

I felt compelled to let everyone know how grateful I was for their support and wanted to almost shout it from the rooftops. The drive within me to say these words was so strong. I felt so passionate, but I was also really scared to make any declaration; still, I knew it was very necessary for me to do it.

As I got ready to make my announcement at the dinner table, my inner critic started its work, saying things like:

- 'What do you think you're doing?'

- 'Who do you think you are?'

- 'They're not going to want to listen to you.'

- 'You are going to make a complete fool of yourself.'

These thoughts were just getting louder and louder. I started to feel terrified as the adrenaline pumped around my system. It was actually quite ridiculous; the feelings were similar to those I would have felt in a situation where I was at risk of being under attack.

My heart started pounding and my throat started to become really dry.

I leaned over to my brother, who was hosting the dinner, and quietly said to him, 'Can you introduce me so I can make a speech after dinner?'

I needed his support with this, as the thought of interrupting everyone talking, and also being loud enough and assertive enough to do it, was something I knew I would find impossible. However, my brother, with his loud and assertive voice and manner, would be able to get everyone's attention.

I stood up on his prompt.

As I opened my mouth to speak, it was like the room disappeared into a haze. My legs felt like they were going to give way underneath me and my voice sounded so strange, like I was speaking underneath a tunnel where the acoustics were really loud. Still, I managed to get the words out and say what I needed to say.

To this day I am so pleased that I did not listen to my inner critic, who was telling me not to do it, as I now know in my conscience that I did the right thing. The thing I really wanted to do. The thing that needed to be said. I was going to stand up and be honest about how I was feeling, regardless of any judgement from myself or anyone else sat around the table.

Of course there was judgement in the room, but I did not let my inner critic be influenced by that.

WHAT'S THIS STEP ALL ABOUT?

The inner critic is that voice inside you that tells you all kinds of information that is negative. This can be very personal, or there can be a practical thing it tells you to do or not to do. This voice is powerful and can influence your decisions. It sends emotional messages that are very powerful and difficult not to respond to. It can also be a voice that resonates in your head on how 'bad' you are or how you have 'failed' in certain areas or situations in your life.

The inner critic is there for a reason: it is a warning system that monitors our activities to make sure we don't walk into high-risk situations. However, we do not actually need to listen to it all of the time, because often it is being too protective. So, even though this step is about 'removing the inner critic', it is actually about learning about your inner critic, understanding it and knowing when to listen to it.

In this section I will break down for you how you can build a relationship with your inner critic so that you can make rational and helpful decisions for yourself based on practicalities and rationality rather than your emotions.

Removing the inner critic comes first in the REBEL method because if that inner voice is not addressed, it will be a block for you. It may even put you off reading any further in this book by telling you that it won't help you, that this method is different and that 'different' is not to be considered or trusted. Or it may tell you that, despite attempts in the past, nothing has worked, so there is no point in trying.

It may tell you that you are a hopeless case or that things are beyond change or your control. These messages may pull you back and stop you from trying, but what you need to know is that they are based on emotion and history, not the reality of today or a practical perspective.

WHY IS THIS IMPORTANT FOR YOU?

This step is particularly important for you as you are already in a dark place in your life, so your inner critic is going to be working overtime to prevent you from feeling worse, but it does not actually know what that involves. So if, for instance, you feel overwhelmed when trying to deal with certain issues, it will tell you not to deal with them and to continue avoiding taking action.

It will also tell you that looking after other people before yourself is the better thing to do because that is what you have always done and what has always been 'safe' for you. Telling people 'No' or perhaps even honestly explaining how you feel may make you feel vulnerable, and that will be an absolute no-no for your inner critic. But this is what you are craving in your life: to put yourself first for once.

The underlying message from your inner critic may be that you are not worthy of a good life. Perhaps you feel you have failed in certain aspects; your inner critic will reinforce this belief and give you negative messages that will prevent you from doing things for yourself. You may feel guilty as a result. Guilt is an emotion linked to a message that you have done something wrong. It is there for a reason but can become unhealthy when it is not valid. Invalid guilt happens when you feel guilty for helping yourself. It does not take account of the fact that if you do not help yourself, you will not be helpful to others any more.

If you do not address your inner critic, the stress will remain, self-blame will remain, and you will continue to feel low. This will prevent you from doing the things you love or want to do. It will prevent you from finding new opportunities and options, resulting in you losing your confidence and all hope of your life moving forward or changing.

If you do not address this inner critic, your negative thinking will continue to dominate your decisions and actions. This will in turn lower your mood and perhaps even cause you to make decisions that are actually more detrimental to your wellbeing. As a result, you will continue to feel the negative emotions of anxiety and depression on a daily basis.

ARIETTA'S STORY

Arietta came from a difficult family background. Her mum struggled with addiction, and her siblings fell into the same problems. She was able to gain some stability in her life through her father, who was divorced from her mother. Arietta had become very successful in her career and was in a stable relationship herself, but she was haunted by beliefs that she did not deserve the good life she had. Her inner critic was extremely powerful and was holding her back from doing anything for herself. One of the decisions she was really struggling with was going into a house purchase. She did not feel that she deserved this; she felt she was not worthy of such a thing.

Arietta would spend so much time going over decisions in her head and overthinking them that she was becoming very stressed. She was feeling frustrated and anxious with her constant ruminating and busy head. Her inner critic was causing her lots of problems, especially in her social life.

Her anxiety was also impacting her husband, as it was affecting their decisions about their life together. Arietta was feeling quite upset and fearful about this and was wondering how much longer he would put up with her incessant indecisiveness. She knew she was spending so much time overthinking situations that sometimes opportunities would pass her by, and she would be left with a feeling of regret before thinking, 'Oh no, I really wanted to do that.'

Arietta so wanted to feel joy in her life, but she felt that this was impossible for her. As she looked at her friends, they seemed so happy and their lives so easy, but hers was not – and that was due to her constant worrying. Sometimes she just found it easier to hide from the world. Her overthinking and inner critical voice, she knew, had made her so serious about things all the time and she never really was able to 'let herself go', something she really desired to do in her life. This really saddened her.

I helped Arietta to remove her inner critic first by challenging the message that she did not deserve things. To challenge their beliefs, I sometimes ask clients to just do something that is against that belief. The belief of Arietta's inner critic was that she did not deserve to do things that were nice for herself. I gave her a first task to buy herself some flowers.

When Arietta came back the next week, she said she had done this but had bought the flowers out of the bargain bucket because it felt too 'spoiling' of herself to buy full-price fresh flowers. When we talked this through together, we decided that this perhaps was not what she needed to do. The following week she bought herself nicer flowers, ones she could really admire and enjoy. It worked! Arietta had started the journey of giving herself permission to do nice things for herself. She felt elated and proud of herself, something she had not felt in ages, and she allowed herself to enjoy the flowers.

The second task was to help her put her own needs in front of others by saying no to situations that she did not want to be in. She received an invitation to a social event that she did not want to attend. As an experiment, and with my support, she said no. On reporting back to me, she said this had felt awkward at first but that she then felt elated at having done it, and she also had a realisation that actually people were not as bothered as she thought they would be, instead appreciating her honesty. She realised how it must have come across when she was not happy doing things but agreed to do them anyway. She realised this behaviour was not only detrimental to herself but to other people as well, as she was perhaps a little moody and unsociable having put herself in these situations.

Arietta recognised that she could only be there for others if she took care of herself first – something she had never done before. She recognised that she was starting to feel so much happier as she quietened and did not listen to her inner critic so much.

We spoke about Arietta's goals and then how she wanted to feel throughout the week. She would look at each action and decide how she should act to enhance a positive feeling within herself. With my help and guidance through this, she started to feel so much better, and she started to take more risks in her life.

She and her husband bought the house; after exploring and challenging all the 'what ifs' in a session, Arietta felt able to take a risk and go for it. Her head had been giving her so many reasons not to do it, and they were mainly ones around her not deserving it. She also stepped out of the comfort zone she had been sitting in at work and took on more responsibility. She was fearful of getting this wrong, but we explored that in a session and decided that, really, the costs she would incur by not moving forward were greater than the benefits of staying in the same place. She became more compassionate with herself, recognising that we can all make mistakes and it is not the end of the world if we do. Arietta said she gained clarity from our work together, as she was not playing through all of the scenarios in her head any more.

One of the sessions covered things we can and cannot control. This has become a large part of Arietta's daily routine: she 'binned' the things on the to-do list that she could not control, freeing up more space in her mind.

Arietta attended one of our retreat workshops that focus intensely on that inner voice. She said that just exploring what she would say to a friend who was struggling and then turning that around to herself in a group exercise really 'hit home' and was extremely powerful for her.

Since Arietta worked with me, she has said that she felt joy for the first time ever in her life. She took another risk and bought a dog, and one day she just burst out laughing in a real 'belly laugh' at something the dog was doing. She said it felt so good and was emotional for her to 'let go' this much and to stop being so serious, as she had been for so many years.

To work with Arietta and to see the transformation within her, the freedom for her to make choices in her life and step into her own power rather than waiting for everyone else to make decisions, was so wonderful. It brought me such joy, as Arietta has so much to give to the world and the people around her but was holding herself back so much. To know she has the freedom to be her now leaves me with such a warm feeling inside. I am as proud of her as she is of herself.

HOW TO REMOVE YOUR INNER CRITIC

Become aware of who your inner critic is

The first step in the process of removing your inner critic is to become aware of it: what it is like, what it says to you and how it affects you. The focus of this step will be to give your inner critic an identity.

Identifying all the characteristics of your inner critic is key. Is it big or small, human or non-human? What does it look like? What is its expression? What is its voice like– quiet, loud, whispering or shouting? Is it wearing any clothes? If so, what are they like?

Having an identity for your inner critic means that you can have a conversation with it, build a relationship with it, and be assertive with it. This may seem counterintuitive, but if we keep pushing our inner critic away, it just keeps coming back louder. It's similar to dealing with a difficult teenager: rather than just telling them to go away, you would need to try to build rapport and trust with them so you could get them to understand where you were coming from. It is the same with your inner critic.

That identity might be a creature or a person or a character; it really does not matter, but an identity is what it needs. My inner critic is a persistent barking dog with quite a ferocious face. This gave me an image, even if it was a little scary. Having this image helped me to identify my inner critic; I even purchased a key-ring figurine of it so that I could talk to it.

"The thing about negative
thoughts is that they
cause negative feelings"

Become aware of what your inner critic says

The next step is to become aware of the key phrases or messages that your inner critic gives you. For example, these might be 'you're not good enough', 'who do you think you are?', 'people won't notice you', or 'people won't want to hear you'. Maybe your inner critic says something more specific to you, perhaps about the way you look, speak or present yourself. You cannot speak back to someone you are trying to ignore, and you need to be clear about the words they are using so that you can argue the points.

Next, it is important to be aware of how your inner critic makes you feel. Whenever you notice that there is a lot of talk going on from your inner critic, check in with how that is making you feel. Is it making you feel good? Probably not. The thing about negative thoughts is that they cause negative feelings. The words of the inner critic are pretty negative and self-condemning, so they will produce some real negative feelings: perhaps depression or anxiety, and feeling stressed, overwhelmed, frustrated, angry, intensely sad or a whole heap of other destructive emotions. Get yourself a feelings chart (just point your camera at the QR code below) and look at it when your inner critic is about. How is it making you feel?

After we have done this, the work begins on removing and reducing your inner critic. We build counterarguments to the words that are being said to you. These can come in the form of self-talk or just repeating to yourself statements opposing the ones that your inner critic is giving you.

This works because the brain naturally needs to work at being positive; it always scans for negativity to protect us, so positive thoughts actually need our conscious effort. The inner critic is there all the time in a way to protect you from messing up, but sometimes it grows so loud that it is now preventing you from doing the things you want to. It has wired your brain, conditioned you to believe it, even though the things it is saying are not necessarily true.

So the positive phrases you come up with to provide a counterargument to your inner critic need to be everywhere: on Post-it notes, in your mind, on your screen saver, in meditations, in your self-talk.

And we can add to the benefits of this positive talk and messages, because our behaviour is so powerful. Whenever we behave differently, the brain responds – so start being kinder to yourself. Start doing nice things for yourself, like you would for someone you love. This sends a powerful message of contradiction to your inner critic who is telling you all this negative stuff. It is giving a message to your brain that you are *not* all those terrible things it calls you, like worthless and not worth listening to. You are contradicting your inner critic by doing something physical that tells you that you are worth it. It could be just giving yourself permission to do something nice for the day for yourself, rather than running around after everyone else. It could be just buying yourself something nice, such as flowers or something else you know you enjoy.

Finally, I would like to speak about something called 'common humanity', discussed in a book by Kristen Neff PhD and Christopher Germer PhD, *The Mindful Self Compassion Workbook: A Proven Way to Accept Yourself, Build Inner Strength and Thrive.*

Remember that we are all common human beings; you are not the only one who is flawed or who has defects or things wrong with you. There is a big wide world out there full of other people who have messed up. They might have similar problems to you, and maybe they have struggled with them in similar ways to you. You are human. No one is perfect. You cannot actually be perfect, because it is impossible to be a perfect human being.

Stop expecting yourself to be perfect – give yourself a break.

It can be helpful sometimes to think about what you would say to a friend who was struggling, perhaps feeling they were not good enough...

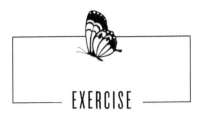

EXERCISE

The point of this exercise is to give your inner critic an identity so that you can talk to it.

Get a piece of paper, or go to the supporting pdf document, and find a pen or some coloured pencils.

To go to the supporting documents and pdf, point your phone's camera at the code below; it will direct you to a page to sign up for access to all the accompanying resources for this book.

If you are able to visualise things in your imagination, do this.

Close your eyes for a moment and think of the worst things you say to yourself. Perhaps imagine the situation where this happens most often. Notice how you are feeling, and hold on to that feeling. Now try to imagine a voice or sound that comes with any harsh words you are hearing in your head. Picture a person, a being, a creature or even an object that would make this kind of noise and even say these words.

Notice everything about this being: their expression, clothes, hair colour, shape, voice tempo and volume, gender. Whatever comes to mind is OK.

Now open your eyes and draw it.

No perfect artistic talent needed; just draw what was in your mind, let it flow onto the paper. If visualisation is difficult for you, that's perfectly understandable (2–5% of the population cannot do this, and only 60% find it easy to do).[1] Instead, you can just draw a picture of what you consider to be an inner critic or your inner critic. Ask yourself: if it had an identity, what would it look like? Colour it in, put an expression on its face, give it a gender (or not, if you prefer), show its size – is it tall or short, fat or thin? Give it a speech bubble illustrating what it is saying, and write some notes underneath about whether it is shouting, whispering or just speaking in an average tone. Give your inner critic a name and write this above the picture.

Now write a sentence underneath your drawing – whether it has come from a visualisation or not – stating what you want to say back to your inner critic. If you are feeling highly creative you could even draw yourself facing your inner critic and speaking to it, so you could then give yourself your own speech bubble.

---

1 https://theconversation.com/aphantasia-explained-some-people-cant-form-mental-pictures-162445

Bonus exercises

1. Think of some counter-statements to your inner
    critical voice, write them down, stick them on Post-its,
    meditate on them, place them on a mirror or on your
    screen saver.

2. Think of something you enjoy or something nice you
    can do for yourself and commit to doing this over the
    next seven days.

SUMMARY

In this chapter we have covered:

✓ Identifying your inner critic and giving it an identity

✓ Noticing how you feel when your inner critic is active

✓ Writing a challenging statement to your inner critic (what you want to say back to it)

✓ Building some positive statements to say to yourself

✓ Finding some positive self-caring activities to do for yourself.

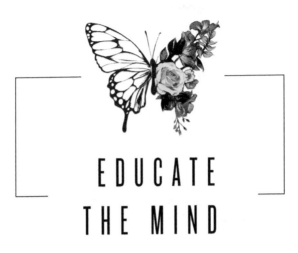

EDUCATE
THE MIND

"Neurons that fire together, wire together."

– DONALD HEBB

I t was my 40th birthday, and my husband had bought me tickets to see Madness, a favourite band of mine when I was a teenager, at the O2 arena. I was excited and thrilled to have this opportunity as we arrived at the venue. I was feeling hyper-excited. We bought some drinks and snacks and headed towards our seats.

It all started really well – I had no idea what was to come. As I started to walk up the metal stairs to our seats, I noticed a really uncomfortable feeling arising in my body. I felt like I was physically going to fall. I looked up; we were already in row V, and our seats were even further up. It felt like I was climbing a precarious rope ladder with an open gorge with a fast-running river underneath about 100 ft down, and the rope was not going to protect me from falling to my death. I was suffering from vertigo for the first time in my life.

I felt overwhelmed; my legs were shaking and I started to crawl on all fours up the metal stairs while trying not to look down through the gaps, which just made me feel physically sick and so anxious. I was concerned that I was not going to be able to attend this concert that my dear husband had brought me to as a birthday treat. I had wanted to see the band live ever since I was a teenager.

I could not overcome the feeling at this point, and there was a strong urge inside me to turn back. I felt like I was going to die. With some encouragement from my husband, I made it on my hands and knees to the seat, turned my body round and placed my bum on the seat, which felt like it was shaking. I took in the area around me, the hundreds of people and the stage far off in the distance, then I happened to glance down. The feeling of panic and fear arose in me again.

Now, I knew logically I could not fall, but the overwhelming sensation that I was going to was unbearable.

At this point in my career I had been learning a lot about the mind and how our thoughts can influence the way we feel. I knew I was having some thoughts subconsciously that were not helping me in this situation, so I decided to take action and train my brain to focus on something other than what it was trying to tell me. Thank goodness I had this awareness.

I recited to myself, 'You are safe. You are not going to fall. It is impossible to fall. There are hundreds of other people here and they are not falling, so the likelihood of you falling is next to nothing.' I repeated this over and over again. Gradually, my feelings of fear and panic started to dissipate and I stopped feeling so shaky.

I had overridden my brain's programming that had been triggered by the height and had begun telling me I was going to fall and that I should get down as quickly as possible, and definitely not to climb any higher. My brain had been trying to protect me, but I had been able to give it new, rational information to counteract its automatic response, which was triggered by fear.

Eventually, I was able to enjoy the concert– in fact, by the end of it, I was actually standing and dancing to the music and able to join in and experience the real joy of being there. It had not been easy, but I had the proof within myself that I could retrain my brain to do something other than what its natural instinct told it to do.

"If we understand why we are feeling the way we are, we put ourselves in a much better position to manage it"

WHAT'S THIS STEP ALL ABOUT?

The E in the REBEL method is all about educating you about your brain and how it works. I will break this chapter down into how we calm our overactive brains, what triggers our brains, what fear really is, the history of our brains, and how to manage negativity and why we have it.

The reason why we need this step next is because knowledge is so important. If we understand why we are feeling the way we are, we put ourselves in a much better position to manage it. In other words, if we know where the leak is coming from, we can fix the plumbing problem.

WHY IS THIS IMPORTANT FOR YOU?

This step is particularly important for you because you are burnt out and overwhelmed but you do not know why. This is causing you to feel hopeless and powerless.

This step is particularly important for you because you are an achiever. You need to know why things are the way they are, and what the solutions are. Once you have this information, you are able to move forward as you have a logical explanation to work with.

It is also particularly important for you because you can really start to understand why you feel the way you do and what part your automatic brain is playing in this feeling. You will be able to stop blaming yourself, because you will understand that so much of how you feel is not your fault.

You will know why you are stuck, and hence you can be kinder to yourself – something you have always wanted, I believe. And even if not, you absolutely deserve to make this change to your life.

You will also learn key techniques in this part of the book to calm your mind and stop the negative thoughts that happen day in, day out. You will get some hope back, because you will start to see how these key techniques can actually help you feel better within yourself.

You will be able to look back at your life and see that the way it has been was perhaps to do with things that were actually not in your control at the time; hence you can forgive yourself, and perhaps others if you feel you want to (this part is certainly not mandatory).

The cost of not understanding how your mind works will be that you will continue to act in the same way and with the same patterns (i.e., you will remain stuck and in your dark hole of negativity, catastrophe and overwhelming feelings). You will have a lack of awareness as to what is automatic in your brain and what you can control about it, so you will continue to blame yourself, leaving you feeling miserable and upset with yourself and your life. You will remain confused and despondent, and your motivation to move forward will remain at a low because you will not get the hope that you can experience from working through this step.

You will continue in patterns of thinking that are destructive to yourself, as you will not understand or know about another way to be. Hence you will lose out on all the opportunity that is ahead of you to feel better and move on to new things. By not working through this step, you will continue to feel hopeless and perhaps even suicidal. You might feel that you cannot go on because, let's face it, life is not great when you are overwhelmed, anxious and depressed all of the time.

ANNIE'S STORY (CONT.)

Annie was an ambitious career woman – a teacher and a medic. She supported her husband throughout his career as an entrepreneur and held the family together in times of financial fluctuation. She had two beautiful grown-up daughters who were ambitious career women themselves and lived in various parts of the world as a result of their successful lives.

There had been a dramatic change in the family situation due to her husband becoming quite unwell, both physically and mentally, and this had started to take a toll on Annie as she tried to facilitate care and support for him. She had been met with a barrage of difficulties, leaving her deflated and despondent at times. The effort she was putting into getting care for him and not getting anywhere left her without her inner resources in the end. She found herself collapsed in a heap, completely numb and with no drive any more when her arrangements backfired as a result of her husband's strong character; he did not want the help that she was trying to put in place for him.

Annie was feeling extremely overwhelmed, to the point that she could not function any more. Her approach in life had always been very much 'get on with a problem and resolve it', but she had found it was not working in this situation; this was, for the first time, a problem that she could not resolve.

Annie also felt abandoned by friends and by services, leaving her helpless. She now felt she needed to just run away from the problem and avoid having to deal with anything. However, this was extremely uncomfortable for her, as it was so unusual for her to feel like this. She had always been quite confident in her ability to 'fix' problems when they arose in life. She had not recognised any problems when dealing with emotions in any other part of her life and felt that she was really struggling for the first time.

One day everything came to a head. Annie felt she had reached the end of her tether; she had no energy left any more to fight. She started to experience feelings of shame: 'could I have done more?' She felt isolated in her problems and could not think straight any more; she was completely overwhelmed. She felt she was in a huge black hole. Annie had lost the ability to be her usual 'functioning' self and had even stronger urges to just run away and give up. This disturbed her immensely, as she had never felt like this before.

Her family were worried about her. Her usual stoic self had gone; she was not coping, and they could see it.

Annie came to me for help. One of the main areas she was really interested in was the practicalities of the mind. I could see that Annie needed to understand that how she was feeling was not her fault. She was experiencing a reaction in her brain, and this was key. I gave Annie compassion for her situation, clarity, insight and knowledge.

Annie had experienced a massively destabilising event in her life, and she really needed this time for her mind to readjust back to a healed state. However, she was not really the type of person who ever rested or took time out for herself. I explained to her how great shocks or difficult events in our lives can cause injury to our brains in the same way as an accident may cause a physical problem in our bodies, such as a broken leg or arm. The advice we are given is to rest the broken bone and to allow it to heal, take the pressure off it; we shouldn't use it for a while and, once the plaster is off, we should do our physiotherapy exercises. It is the same with our brain after we experience a difficult event or a shock: we need to rest it for a while, then do our exercises to heal the injury, so to speak.

Annie started to get the idea of putting herself first and taking care of her emotional needs. I believe it was a relief for her to talk through how she was feeling – after all, this is something we all need to do. It's important to find someone we can talk to when difficult times strike. Annie started to extract some positive affirmations– statements that were positive towards herself, things she could say to herself– from our work together. She also added into her daily routine some activities to bring positivity into her life. This was the opposite of what she had been experiencing, healing her very negative mindset, which had become reinforced through no fault of her own but through her brain trying to cope with the very difficult situation she had found herself in.

Annie came to one of my online workshops; this one was on resilience. In this course we learnt about a part of the brain that responds to stress and stores information but then re-releases it in similar situations in a way that is out of our control.

While in this workshop, Annie saw that there had been some previous 'conditioning' to her brain. She had become accustomed to certain situations throughout her life, but she was struggling to react in a different way today, which was something she needed to do.

By understanding this conditioning of her mind, Annie was able to do things differently, such as checking things out with other people, believing in herself and not responding to situations in her 'old' way but training her brain to use a new reaction. This was not easy for her and caused some frustration, but she persevered and soon started to see the results.

We spoke about SIDs – 'seemingly inconsequential decisions'. These are the decisions we can make based on previous conditioning of our minds that can lead us into old patterns or more difficulty – a bit like the addict who is trying to stop using drugs but subconsciously decides to walk to the shop via the route that takes him past his dealer's house. We make decisions like this all the time, as our brain operates automatically, leading us to always walk the same way to the shop or avoid certain things because they may have caused us pain in the past. Quite often, we don't even know we are doing it. The brain is just programmed on repeat. Sometimes we might need to place boundaries with other people in our lives, recognising that we need to do things differently; saying 'No' instead of our usual 'Yes' can be so important as a way to make changes. Until we realise that we are automatically saying 'Yes', though (and this may be due to previous experiences or 'programming'), it is hard to move forward, as there will always be that internal drive to behave the same way we have always done.

Through self-belief, self-compassion and retraining her brain – as well as allowing it to rest – Annie started to feel less overwhelmed. The exercises in our sessions made her feel more able to cope, too, but she also started to recognise her limitations. This was a massive step for Annie, as she had always held great pride in her abilities to cope with difficult situations— which she had always done, but this one was different and had pushed her to her limit.

This was a good thing. Annie was now able to be kinder to herself, which in turn removed the feelings of shame. As she started to understand what had happened with her brain and the conditioning she had experienced throughout her life, she was able to make better choices and decisions. They were ones that supported her wellbeing and also meant she was able to 'let go' of situations she could not control. This was really difficult for her, but knowing that it was essential for her wellbeing drove her forward.

The results were clear: she started to feel calmer, accepting the situation she had found herself in and finding more clarity in her thinking again. She also found herself doing more daily self-care, such as journaling, yoga and other activities that helped her become calmer.

Annie was such a pleasure to work with. She journaled all her feelings throughout our journey together and, as she read some of her writings back to me, I recognised the power of this work and how it can really help someone to come out of a dark place in their lives. The fact that she received hope gave me such a beautiful image of her life ahead of her– the one she thought was over. The joy she could experience in her own life became apparent as she was able to 'let go' of her need to resolve the difficulties she had experienced and enjoy her life as it was. I loved working with Annie, seeing someone find hope when all there had been was darkness. After all, I can so relate to that journey. It brings me joy to see others find their path too.

HOW TO EDUCATE YOUR MIND

Get aware

The first step in this process is to educate yourself about your brain and understand what goes on inside it. Here are three really useful points about the brain:

1. The brain naturally scans for negatives, so you need to work to retrain your brain to be more positive. This function is only the brain automatically trying to help us by scanning for dangers, areas we may be making mistakes in, or people we need to be wary of. Our brains have always done this to keep us safe, ever since prehistoric times. The problem with this can be intense personal criticism for making mistakes (our brain going into a real negative place when we are about to take risks that can essentially help us to move forward – resistance) and a lack of trust in others.

2. What fires together, wires together. If you have been in a negative space and thought processes for a while, your brain will be much more used to sending you more negative thoughts than positive ones, so this is what it will continue to do until it starts to rewire.

3. Sometimes there are things that 'stick' in our brains. These can be learned behaviours (conditionings), messages from other people consistently over time (conditionings) or traumatic experiences. Traumatic experiences are stored in a different part of the brain (the emotional brain); this is the part that responds to triggers. For example, a song may give you the feeling of something traumatic that happened, or a person's look or mannerisms may trigger an emotional feeling of someone who traumatised you in the past. This is the brain doing its job, warning you that you may be in danger again.

Being aware of the way your brain works – based on some of your experiences, your history and also the fact you are a human being – is key as a first step. None of this is your fault, because your brain really does do things on its own, despite your attempts to will it not to. Fear can come up at any time and is an emotional reaction to triggers or a response from your brain because it thinks you are in danger. In prehistoric times our brains were programmed to produce a stress response: more energy; a temporary draining of blood from non-essential functions; an increase in adrenaline; sweating, shaking, alertness and readiness to deal with a threat. Today this part of our brain is still in operation, and the slightest fear or perceived danger can trigger this 'fear' response automatically.

Now that you have this awareness, the next step is to start retraining your brain.

There are three key things you can do to start to rewire your brain:

- Mindfulness

- Breathwork

- Gratitude lists

All of these things help to calm the brain and send a counteracting message to your 'high-alert' brain that all is well.

Start to learn about mindfulness

Mindfulness helps you to focus on what really is happening and not on what you believe is happening, what you have experienced in the past, or what you are fearful of for the future. Mindfulness can be as simple as going for walks and noticing the trees or the sky. It can be doing a creative activity, such as making something, or it can be a martial art or yoga. When you are practising mindfulness, the parasympathetic nervous system kicks in. This is also known as the 'rest and restore' mechanism. During this time, the hormones produced in the fight-or-flight response reduce, and your system can be restored to a normal state. This is essential for mental wellbeing.

Focus on your breathing

(Please remember that this is only to be used if you do not suffer from panic attacks from this kind of approach.)

Noticing your breath and focusing on it calms everything down in your brain – again, it is a mindful exercise, but it also has other benefits for your energy levels as your oxygen level increases. Focusing on your breath and slowing your breathing down helps to reprogramme the brain, telling it there is no danger. A useful way to do this is to follow your breath flowing in and out of your mouth or nose, notice your diaphragm rising and falling, and put your hands on your belly, feeling it rise and fall as you breathe. Just concentrate on that. Try it now while you are sitting reading or listening to this book (but not if you are driving).

Gratitude

Gratitude lists help you to focus on the positive things in your life. There will always be something to be grateful for, even if it is just the fact that you have food to eat or a roof over your head. However, as I said earlier, the brain automatically focuses on what is lacking as part of its prehistoric survival strategy for us.

Reinforcing the positives in your life will start to change your brain's focus. Like a computer, what you feed into it will determine what comes back out of it. There is a saying 'neurons that fire together, wire together', first said by neuropsychologist Donald Hebb in 1949[2]. His discovery was that as neurons (cells which transmit the electrical signals in the brain) operate more, they encourage other neurons in the brain to operate in the same way. It's a bit like 'following the crowd'. More will become attached the more there are. We could liken this to a movement that perhaps starts as an idea, and then more people latch onto it and start using it.

---

2 https://neurosciencenews.com/wire-fire-neurons-19835

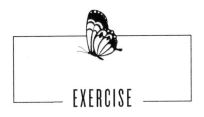

EXERCISE

Gratitude diaries

This exercise is about increasing the positive wiring of your brain to help you feel better and to retrain the way you think– which is absolutely possible– so that you can start to be more positive. Remember: what fires together wires together.

Get a notebook or a piece of paper, or use the notes app on your phone or the page in the workbook PDF by following the QR code below for resources. Write down seven things you are grateful for. This is the beginning of your gratitude diary.

If you would like to continue this exercise for longer, then go to my resources page via the QR code, where you can access my 10-day gratitude challenge.

SUMMARY

In this chapter we have covered:

✓ The neuroscience of the brain, brain conditioning and the prehistoric brain's safety mechanism

✓ How using mindfulness can help to rewire the brain, and what we mean by 'mindfulness'

✓ How breathing can simply calm down the fight-or-flight brain response

✓ Using gratitude to rewire the brain's negativity

✓ Further exercises you can do to continue with the great journey of rewiring your brain.

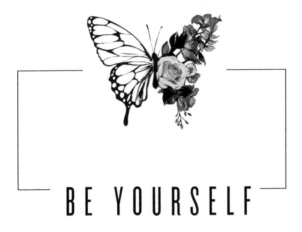

BE YOURSELF

"Knowing yourself is the beginning

of all wisdom."

– ARISTOTLE

I n 2017 I was let go from my job.

In the back of my mind, working for other people had been discouraging me from truly being me, but I had not had the courage to allow that to come through until this point. It was almost as if I was given this opportunity specifically in order for this to happen.

Let me just take you back to an earlier chapter, where we met Vanessa. Throughout my life I have been learning about myself, and this has brought me to today, where I mostly understand who I am, what I need in life and therefore have gained some ability to live in alignment with who I am.

As I stated in that previous chapter, there were three points in my life when I made significant shifts in discovering who I was as a person and hence moved towards being more authentically me. The first was after my bad car accident in 1998, when I had lots of time laid up recovering from some quite serious injuries. During this time, I enrolled on a counselling course. It was a revelation. I discovered I had choices in my life, something I had not realised before. I realised I could change my life if I wanted to, even though I was feeling pretty hopeless, negative and overwhelmed at the time. I also learnt I could be myself and that if I was not happy with things in life, I could change them. Consequently, I left the relationship with my children's father.

The second point was in 2008, when I was ill for a period with swine flu. I was in a high-pressure job at the time and working many hours. Life at home was not easy. I was constantly stressed and quite depressed. Things just did not seem right. I had started taking some herbal supplements to manage my depression, but I was waking up feeling so dark and bleak every morning. I was thinking, 'Is this it? Is this what my life has become?' Even though I was away from the chains of addiction, my life was not right. I felt dissatisfied, incomplete, like I was living a life that other people felt I should live but that I did not like myself. I was constantly anxious about sharing my voice and truth, and felt I was just swaying from one crisis to the next in my life.

During this time, I started to look at some coaching tools. I came across some that helped me to understand what I wanted in my life and how I could implement them. I learnt what my values were, and aimed towards living in alignment with them. This was a process, but once I knew what my values were – connection, responsibility and growth – and once I started making sure that everything I did in life was in alignment with them, I found life became a lot more fulfilling.

The last period was in 2018 when I was launching into my business. Having been let go by my company, as I mentioned above, I was able to truly become me. I explored so many aspects of myself, using coaching tools and personality questionnaires. I explored crystal healing, colour therapy, meditation, yoga, feng shui and energy healing. I gained a coaching qualification. Most importantly, I changed my life significantly to correlate with everything that I now knew was me. I changed things at home. I allowed myself to explore lifelong ambitions, one of them being to scuba dive, and I made a commitment to stop pleasing people and not to worry what other people thought of me. It was truly freeing, and I can quite honestly say it is the best thing I have done for my mental health.

WHAT'S THIS STEP ALL ABOUT?

This step is all about being truly in alignment with yourself and being authentic to who you are. It is about saying no to the things you don't want or need in your life. It is about saying yes to the things you do want and need in your life. It is about placing boundaries in your life, stopping people-pleasing and stopping worrying about what others may think. It is also about developing compassion for yourself and letting go of being so harsh on yourself, accepting who you are and letting go of those 'shoulds' in life that we take on so often and feel we have to fulfil.

The reason why this step comes here is that you now have an opportunity to put into action some of the things you learnt in the first two steps. By following this step now, you really start to firm up your progress and your moving forward. By understanding your real, true and authentic wants and needs and putting them into practice, you can build some hope of a better future, because you will be putting your needs first more often. This will feel good. I can guarantee that it will prompt you to continue with this journey.

WHY IS THIS IMPORTANT FOR YOU?

This step is particularly important for you because, probably for the first time in your life, you have an opportunity ahead of you to be truly you. You may not believe this at this point, and you will feel as if other factors (e.g., people and situations) are preventing this. However, this is not the truth. You *can* be you, but perhaps your first task is to find out who you really are. You have spent so many years looking after other people or perhaps chasing a career that you have never had the opportunity or need to broach this question.

You are never too old to do this.

You may discover new activities or delights in your life as you go on this journey of discovery. A sense of newness and adventure, however small, is so good for our mental wellbeing.

Over the years, you may have felt unheard or neglected, but now you have the opportunity to hear yourself and respond to the things you say. Once you know what your needs are and what fulfils you, you can do more of it, which will massively help your mental health.

With self-acceptance comes the ability to let go of the past and to look to the future. Living in regret is futile.

The greatest benefit for you will be the peace of mind that will come with being you. A real sense of calm will come over you, others will be unable to phase you so much, and you will have less need for all those negative thoughts and worries. You may not need to worry about other people any more. You can choose to worry about them, but that will be something you will be much more in control of, and it will be your choice.

If you do not bring this step into your life, then you may continue to be resentful with others and yourself; you will continue to ruminate on worry, guilt and self-pity. This will cause you to continue to feel miserable and it will impact your relationships with others, as well as your already shattered faith in humanity. Anger and frustration will still be present in your life and will impact upon you.

You will also continue to be overwhelmed and have too much on your plate, because you will not take the time to scale everything back to what is really important for you in life. When you are overwhelmed, you feel you cannot cope, and this will not go away if you do not work through this step of the programme. The overwhelm and inability to cope will continue to contribute to your stagnation and lack of motivation, paralysing you and preventing you from seeing a way forward. In the long term, this will lead to continued anxiety and depression and perhaps feelings of hopelessness or even not wanting to be here any more.

NAOMI'S STORY

Naomi came to me for help early last year. She was exhausted, felt she had lost focus in her life and was feeling extremely frustrated with her life.

She was aware that she had a difficult history as both her parents had been alcoholics. This, she said, was impacting her on a daily basis and she was having frequent bad dreams, even though it had been many years since she had left home.

As a child she had taken on the role of caring for her parents and had also acted as mediator during their conflicts and arguments. She had found herself keeping the peace or making the environment better, hiding the evidence from the outside world so that no one knew and it remained the family secret.

She would also just retreat to her room, alone and unsupported, when things became bad.

Naomi also had come to realise that making decisions was really difficult for her. She always had her parents, and her background 'duty of care' to them, on her mind. She found herself in overwhelm and fear so often.

The other thing was that Naomi found it extremely difficult to express her needs to others when she knew things were not right. She would become overwhelmed and find herself paralysed, unable to take any action, and then this would make her feel hopeless, depressed and enveloped in so much self-doubt.

The two of us explored Naomi's fears in her sessions and discussed the roles that her upbringing had imprinted on her. Through my help and knowledge around family dynamics in addiction, Naomi was able to see how she had become the 'caretaker' in the family. We explored and identified together how each of her behaviours today – the paralysis, the difficulty making decisions, the overwhelm – were rooted back in her childhood role.

Then I worked with Naomi, teaching her new techniques to identify her needs and then to take actions to put her needs first. This was not an easy process and, if you can relate at all, I am sure you recognise how difficult putting yourself first can be when you have had a lifetime of caring for others. Naomi learnt what her values were and also what her strongest drivers were in her behaviour, how both her values and her drivers impacted who she was, and how she interacted with the world and others.

The other area Naomi was struggling with involved some cultural expectations associated with the country from which she originated. She still felt the pressure to follow the lifestyle choices of her home country.

As Naomi started to identify her own needs, she was able to make peace with her difference and she was able to let go of the cultural 'shoulds'. This process came only through the self-acceptance work we did, exploring her own qualities, affirming them and taking steps in her behaviour that were aligned with who she truly is. She needed a lot of support from me in this first step as her self-doubt and overwhelm would often come in and take over, but staying focused on the 'right' decision– the one that serves her and gives her positive feelings– really helped. Working out what this was took some time, but we got there in the end. There were tears and revelations, but throughout a period of three months, including six sessions and a three-day retreat, Naomi started to feel more confident and free within herself.

Naomi moved to a new home with a friend she felt comfortable with. Previously she had been living in a shared house with people she felt she 'should' be comfortable with but, in fact, their negative behaviour was really affecting her. Naomi was able to conserve her energy by doing this, as she was no longer help-ing others sort out their problems in her home envi-ronment. This was something she had slipped into so naturally, even though it was destructive to her, as a result of the family dynamic she had come from.

I often say to my clients that it is so easy to put on that old pair of slippers that are worn out and comfort-able, although they really are not good for your health.

137

New slippers may feel uncomfortable to begin with, but they will also make you feel clean and fresh. They will support you better and will help you shine rather than being dull and stained.

Naomi started to feel so much better within herself; she felt happy and adopted the phrase 'Yes, I can'. This gave her permission to do things for herself, something that was entirely alien to her. She said she now felt able to trust herself and that the overwhelming and obsessive self-doubt had slipped away. Of course, it would come back on occasions, but she had the tools now to identify it and work through it, pushing it to the side so she could move forward.

Naomi started to practise mindfulness on a daily basis. I had taught her all the elements of mindfulness, and its benefits in different situations, throughout our time together. This helped her to cope in situations where she felt overwhelmed, and to take a step back.

She started to feel really proud of herself as she pushed through with changes in her life, working towards her goals free of guilt and conflicting thoughts. Naomi really came to understand who she was and was able to 'be herself', and so her mental health improved immensely. She felt happy and content, at peace when making decisions in her life and firm in what she wanted, with no self-doubt or internal conflict. Her relationships improved so much as a result.

After the three months, Naomi was quite honestly a changed and transformed person who now completely understood her limitations, herself and her needs. She was able to give herself permission to be herself and was behaving in a completely new way in her life. The result for her was so thrilling.

HOW TO BE YOURSELF

Identify your needs

The first part of this step is to find out what your needs, your wants and your desires are. There are a few ways to do this and, firstly, once you have started to self-care, removed the inner critic and understood that default position of your brain's programming, then you are free to build the person you truly are and want to be.

This step is not about inventing a new personality or having unrealistic ideas about being someone who is really not you; it is about aligning yourself with who you really are. This is why this part comes after the first two steps, because part of this process involves acceptance of who you are. This truly is an incredible process, and the combination of accepting yourself and moving into your truth will ensure that you will feel so free and so empowered.

Everyone has different values in life. Firstly, you need to find out what yours are. You probably have some idea, but completing an exercise to help you find this out can be really helpful. This is certainly what I did, and it really helped me.

Start saying no

The second part is then to start saying no to things that are not in alignment with your values, and yes to things that are.

You should place boundaries in those areas of your life where you know your energy is getting wasted, and stop worrying so much about what other people think. By this I really mean that if people are not helping you be in alignment with your values, then you should not spend so much time with them. Your recovery is too important not to do this.

My values are connection, growth and responsibility. I spent so much of my life living out of alignment with these values. I was not taking responsibility in my life, and I was actually isolating myself from other people. To change this behaviour, I had to say no to the inner critic that was telling me people would not want to connect with me because I had nothing to say.

Say, for instance, that your value is justice. This is an area you may need to pursue if there is an injustice in your life. By doing this, you are saying no to allowing injustices in your life. Similarly, if your value is empathy and you find yourself surrounded by people who are not empathic, then you need to say no to these people being in your life.

Here are some examples of saying yes to things that are in alignment with your values. Being more in nature, if that is your value. Allowing yourself to love, if this is a value, and finding areas where you can experience this value. If your value is work, then it is important to say yes to work that you really enjoy.

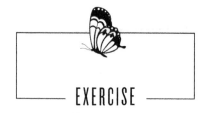

EXERCISE

"It is never too late to be what you might have been."

– GEORGE ELIOT

The first exercise is for you to find out what your values are (go to the pdf worksheet via the QR code below). Spend some time working on this. Before you do this exercise, just sit quietly for five minutes, focusing on your breath or allowing your mind to settle if you can. This will allow you to focus and to get the clarity you need.

The point of this exercise is for you to know what you need to work towards. It will help you to have a clear vision of the path ahead of you and what needs to change. Be easy on yourself, though; you do not have to change all of this overnight.

Do remember also that there will be conditioning from step two that will pop up as you make these changes. Your brain will start to scream out, 'This is not how we have always done things!' Your brain does not like changes in behaviour because it resists going out of the comfort zone that you have been in, but you need to challenge this reaction. Do be compassionate with yourself about this, though, because the feelings will be strong to go back to your old ways. Notice your resistance, acknowledge it and talk to yourself gently about the long-term goals of happiness and peace of mind you are working towards.

Then work out what your values are, making sure you pick three. These are who you truly are. Notice the feeling as you think about these values – you will know what feels right. Now you are ready to move forward slowly in your life, looking at what is in alignment and what is not.

Think of five areas in your life that do not feel right for you, and ask yourself:

- What is the area?

- What value is not being met?

- What needs to change?

- What one thing can you do this week to align with your values?

- What one thing can you do this month to align with your values?

- What one thing can you do this year to align with your values?

SUMMARY

In this chapter we have covered:

✓ Being in alignment with who you are

✓ Your values

✓ Saying no

✓ Saying yes

✓ Placing boundaries in your life

✓ Stopping the people-pleasing and the worrying about what others think

✓ Being easy on yourself.

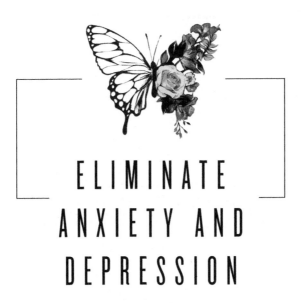

ELIMINATE ANXIETY AND DEPRESSION

"Once your mindset changes, everything on the outside will change along with it."

– STEVE MARABOLI

I n 2017, when I was let go from my job, I was not expecting it. I was told I needed to leave that day, and it came as a huge shock. At the time, it was devastating; it felt catastrophic and I was so overwhelmed with shock and disappointment that I felt extremely anxious about what I was going to do. It was the first time in 12 years that I had been without steady employment. I was reliant on the monthly salary for all my needs: mortgage, household bills, supporting family members. I felt quite depressed and hopeless.

This was a difficult time in my life. I decided that the best way forward was to set up my own business, although I had no idea whether I could make it. When I was starting this business, I would cry a lot. I was full of uncertainty and self-doubt. I woke up feeling depressed and anxious, often on a daily basis.

In my attempts to learn how to run my own business, I came across a business coach called Carl Brooks. I decided to attend a retreat, where I was going to learn how to run a coaching business. On this retreat, where there were just four of us, I learnt key messages about being yourself, but I was also introduced to yoga and meditation.

I needed to work on my 'I can't' mindset. It was powerful at this time. As I said, I was full of self-doubt and fear. I had lots of underlying beliefs that had been with me since I was a child, and I needed to work through all of them. I was full of fear but had to keep pushing through. So I took risks and I embraced failure as part of the journey. I needed coaching and help with this, though.

Following this retreat, I started to learn about lots of resources from the other ladies who had joined me; these included feng shui, colour therapy and energy healing. I also started to understand how meditation and mindfulness helped my mood, and especially how yoga helped me.

I have always suffered with mood swings in my life. However, I can quite honestly say that, now that I use a combination of all these tools, my life has become free of anxiety and depression. Don't get me wrong; I do still get down, but I now know that giving in to a negative mind-set and not facing my fears or not practising my self-care routine will soon leave me slipping back into anxiety and depression.

I do get anxious when having to speak in public, and I do get depressed sometimes. You know that one where you wake up at 3am with a really dark feeling? I get up, I meditate, I journal my feelings and thoughts, and I use all of the tools that I have learnt over the last few years– and I can honestly say that I have eliminated my anxiety and depression and can control my mood now.

These are not the only tools I use. I have learnt to recognise where my difficult feelings come from and have learnt to accept them. Indeed, with acceptance comes the ability to move forward. I don't feel I am fighting my demons any more. Eliminating my anxiety and depression involves a daily routine of self-care. However, now I know what it is that I need, I can put the tools in place.

The routine is like dental hygiene – mental hygiene, if you like. I also have different tools for different problems. Knowledge, acceptance and then action is everything for me.

- Knowledge: understanding why I am struggling. Is my brain doing something automatically for me? Am I believing some negative thoughts? Am I not aligned with myself and my life's purpose? Am I practising daily mental health self-care?

- Acceptance: accepting circumstances and people I cannot change, letting go of what I can't control and controlling what I can.

- Action: practising self-care, facing fears, asking for help, actively changing my mindset and challenging the automatic thinking that comes from my prehistoric safety-seeking brain.

WHAT'S THIS STEP ALL ABOUT?

This step is about eliminating your underlying anxiety and depression. I will help you to understand why you might feel depressed or anxious in particular circumstances or situations. I will give you techniques to manage anxiety and techniques to manage depression. I will show you how to change your mindset on a daily basis. I will help you work through fear of any changes. You will gain tools for managing your self-care, your health and your mental wellbeing, and tools to help with sleep.

Building on what we have learnt in the previous steps, this step is the maintenance step. It is a toolkit of all the things you can do to manage your anxiety, depression and your moods. This in turn will enhance your experience of life and how you feel about it.

This step secures your longer-term recovery and prevents relapse back into the way you have been feeling recently. You will understand how creativity, journaling and meditation can be your saviours. You will learn how to stay in tune with yourself and your needs so you do not go off track.

Eliminating your anxiety and depression is so import-ant because you can have the quality of life that you so deserve. You have worked hard, and it is important that the time you have left here is not clouded by problems with your mental health.

This step is all about you taking better care of your-self, but primarily it is about taking care of your mental wellbeing. By working through this step, you will continue to have better motivation to try new things, you will not get pulled back down into the dark hole you have been in, and you will have flexibility and coping strategies and skills to deal with those curveballs that life can throw at us. Not having mood swings, anxiety or depression, and having the tools to eliminate them from your life, will naturally give you peace of mind. You will lose the worry about being able to cope in particular situations. You may feel fear of trying new things, but you will do them because you will want to move towards happiness and peace of mind and will know what gives you that. You will be able to let the past be the past and not let it drag you down today.

WHY IS THIS IMPORTANT FOR YOU?

You will understand what your blocks are and therefore know when to get help or what tools you can use to get through them and move on to the next step. You may find yourself taking some steps forward and then a few back at this point, but you now have the tools and the understanding to deal with them as blips rather than things getting progressively worse.

By skipping this step, you will continue to feel unmotivated, which leads to feeling unfulfilled in life, leaving you feeling despondent, hopeless and depressed. You may risk slipping back, repeating how you have been feeling recently. Feeling the same things is inevitable, but you have a choice now in this step to move forward or slip back. If you do not pay attention to this step, this may have a negative impact on your relationships, bringing you sadness and regret at this point in your life.

By not moving forward with this, you will remain stuck as you are in the patterns you have established over many years. You may even continue to feel worse unless you face this.

JULIE'S STORY

Julie had been having anxiety attacks for a couple of years. Lately, prior to meeting me, these had turned into panic attacks and had become quite frequent. She was also experiencing depression, which would leave her unable to get out of bed for three or four days in a row.

Julie felt like she was going crazy; she was so depressed and anxious that it had started to affect her physically. She was experiencing lots of feelings of shame, guilt and sadness. In addition, she had been suffering with persistent back pain for over a year, which was preventing her from pursuing her career, so she was unable to work. Julie was also getting stomach pain that would come on with the anxiety, which was crippling and debilitating for her and left her in a vicious cycle of not being able to work or do activities that she knew were good for her, such as exercise. Her previous busy, energetic life had become non-existent and she had lost all confidence, feeling so low and depressed most of the time that it left her unable to function.

She was struggling with resentments, especially towards her mother, who she felt had not supported her in her life. Julie was also extremely judgemental towards herself about anything, even washing the dishes!

She said that judgements from people, especially those close to her, would 'eat her alive'.

Julie lacked the motivation to do the things she felt she should be doing. This was impacting upon her relationship with her partner and left her feeling guilty about her interactions with her children. She hated them seeing her so upset all the time; she was crying constantly and could not stop the tears coming at frequent points throughout the day. The smallest of tasks would overwhelm her and then she would be wracked with guilt, persecuting herself over feelings of being useless. She could not get the thoughts of 'what's wrong with me?' out of her mind. Julie did not want to go onto medication but knew she needed to do something, as it felt like her life had ended.

She was having frequent disturbingly bad negative thoughts and was feeling so angry and on edge most of the time, which caused her to have arguments with her husband. This would then trigger her into thinking and feeling that she was a really bad person. All of this meant that she was panicking about upcoming family events and did not feel that she could face family and friends.

Initially, we looked at Julie's goals for the therapy and broke these down to work on one at a time. Julie's belief system about herself was very negative, and this was increasing her anxiety and depression. Thoughts like 'I am not good enough' were plaguing her daily.

I showed her some cognitive behavioural techniques to manage her thoughts. These also helped her to have more self-acceptance and compassion for herself about what she had been through in her past. She had not had an easy life, with bad relationships and a mother who had abandoned her.

We incorporated lots of meditation techniques into Julie's sessions. One particular meditation took Julie to a place where she met her inner child at various points in her life and was able to heal the hurt and the feelings of expectation she had placed on herself.

Through meditation I helped her to 'cut the cords' of resentment she had with her mother and to find more of the acceptance that she craved but was unable to get from her mother. This again left her with more acceptance, hence removing the feelings of frustration and anger that were plaguing her mind and making her feel quite crazy.

We used mindfulness with her feelings and her thoughts, helping her to manage the waves that came and went. We used grounding techniques (a form of meditation) to help her cope when she was feeling overwhelmed, and coping strategies to deal with a 'bad day'.

Julie started to practise some compassion for her body, such as yoga and stretching, walking in nature or just allowing herself the space to sit and meditate and be calm. She started to listen to her body more and not fight when she felt unwell. All of this helped her depression. Within six months of working with me she was so much happier and was pain-free in both her stomach and her back. (Disclaimer here: I never advised Julie at any point to not get other factors checked out with her doctor in regard to her stomach and back pain.)

As a result of the work we did together and the healthy wellbeing habits she formed, Julie gained more understanding of her thoughts and of what was going on in her body; for instance, how her body was indicative of how she was feeling. She was able to recognise the link between stress and her stomach aches, and found that her inner critic was basically gone.

She was also able to understand her feelings and allow herself to have them. Understanding her own emotions was something she had never been able to do before. She said that she had me in her head saying, 'Is this really important? Perhaps you can let this go?' She was able to take the pressure off herself and hence felt so much calmer by using the meditation skills that we had practised together.

As a result, Julie was less angry and was able to be calmer, not on edge all the time. She spoke about how she was feeling more and worrying less about burdening others by expressing her feelings when she needed to; hence the small things that led to big explosions of anger were not building up in the same way. She found and used other physical ways to manage her anger, such as working out or boxing.

She stopped getting so upset and down over little things, finding hope and excitement instead. In fact, she was starting to look forward to what was to come in her life. She recognised that the way she viewed things and her life had completely shifted for her.

Julie was able to understand that some of the fears in her relationship were actually her husband's, and how that impacted her. They began talking more. Julie recognised that she needed to take her husband's feelings into consideration too, something she had been unable to do previously as she had been so overwhelmed with her own insecurity and her doubt that he was being loving enough. She had been taking on too much responsibility for his feelings, and realised how this was affecting her energy as well as taking her back to thinking about past relationships that had been difficult.

She learnt skills with me to protect herself and to not become overwhelmed in these situations. Through this, she gained insight into her relationship with her mum and the dynamic she had with her. She understood that her mum was a bit of a rescuer and did not affirm her progress. Julie was able to let go of the anger that she had with her mum. Her behaviour changed around her, and she stopped some of the contact. She recognised that her feelings around her mum were valid and was able to come to terms with this and not blame herself any more.

She declared, 'I have stopped thinking that I am the crazy one.'

Julie recognised that a lot of the judgements she made were self-inflicted; she started to remember conversations and how they had not been so full of the criticism she had perceived previously. Again, this was a massive change in mindset and perspective. This helped her to really reduce that sense that she was not good enough.

With my help, Julie recognised changes in her behaviours and mindset with a lot more self-acceptance. She was able to take some of the pressure off herself to always have a purpose, so she was being less harsh on herself about the position she was in currently in her life. She was able to connect with joy rather than judgement, to stop overthinking things that seemed difficult and start to 'just do' things if she wanted to do them, like going for a walk or doing yoga. This in turn prevented self-blame and brought in more feelings of being proud of herself, hence increasing her motivation.

Her back pain had gone completely after three months of us working together. This really happened after a real eye-opening session with me where she was able to self-heal the pain through meditation. She continued to use yoga to manage her physical pain and she found that she had the ability to self-heal her pain.

She also took up painting and photography to express her feelings, as writing and journaling were difficult for her. This creative outlet really helped her to feel her emotions and to express herself; hence the overwhelm was reduced for her. She felt more emotionally balanced on a daily basis.

I absolutely loved working with Julie and seeing the changes in her and the freedom that she experiences now, finding herself free from the daily effects of anxiety and depression on her mind and body.

HOW TO ELIMINATE ANXIETY AND DEPRESSION

This is a key step to managing your anxiety and depression. Even as you complete the steps above, you may still experience those feelings, but you really are on a good road to tackling them. Still, remember the conditioning we spoke about in step two that will still be there?

This step is all about developing tools to manage your symptoms.

These will also be quite individual to you. Some of these might already have come to light for you; for instance, if health is a value of yours, healthy eating and exercise may be key to your ongoing recovery. If your value is creativity, then having time out to do creative things may be key to your recovery.

Work on your mindset

You will need to manage your thinking. Our thinking is directly related to how we feel, so negative and self-destructive thinking acts as a massive block, as we saw in step one when we learned about our inner critic and its negative messages.

A great part of this step is to work on your mindset, and to find out whether you have a growth or a fixed mindset. You may find that in some areas you have a growth mindset but in others you are definitely fixed. Below is an explanation of each of the different mindsets that we can have.

A growth mindset helps you to focus on the positives, to be more flexible, to see possibility. You will be more of a 'cup half full' person and will also be able to celebrate other people's achievements rather than feeling resentful about the things that they have and you don't.

A fixed mindset is often full of statements like 'I can't', 'It's useless', 'I am too unwell', 'This won't work for me', 'I am a hopeless case', 'This has gone too far, and I cannot change now'. These types of statements and mindsets will just prevent you from moving forward. They leave you in a position where trying seems pointless– but if you do not try, then things cannot move forward.

To work on your anxiety and depression, you need to work on your mindset. If you have a fixed mindset about something, see how you can turn this into a growth mindset and start saying the relevant statement to yourself frequently. Even write down the growth mindset somewhere and read it every day.

Work on your fears

The second step is to work on your fears, because fear holds you back. Often with change there will be fear – this is only natural, but too much fear causes anxiety, and not addressing our fears but staying safe where we are causes depression. Therefore, fear needs to be faced.

You may worry about taking the steps you need to take through a fear of being rejected, which is especially common if you are trying to be authentically you for the first time. People may reject you, but do you really want them in your life if they are only in it because of a version of yourself that is not you?

You may be afraid of your own feelings. After all, change can bring feelings – feelings of uncertainty, feelings of being out of control, feelings of loss – and we need to face these to address our anxiety and depression. Think of one small thing you can do today to face your fears and be authentic to yourself.

A common fear is a fear of being alone. This can be an overwhelming feeling, especially if you are going through a relationship break-up or a bereavement or loss. Be aware of how you might continue to please others because you fear rejection from them. However, also be aware that this behaviour will not help your anxiety and depression. Taking risks is a part of recovery and growth.

I know you can do this! I have your back and, believe me, you will find yourself with a heap of new people in your life when you start to be more confident and genuine with yourself. When you have your motivation back, you will make new friends– people who are good for you and have your interests at heart.

Work on your lifestyle

The third step is to implement some healthy habits for your wellbeing:

- Giving up or reducing alcohol consumption

- Taking more walks

- Getting time for you

- Making a space that is yours in your home where you find peace

- Eating more healthily

- Exercising (very good if you have experienced trauma in your life)

- Getting better sleep

- Letting go of commitments

- Letting go of people

- Changing jobs

- Moving

- Saying no to things you don't want in life

- Saying yes to things you do want in life.

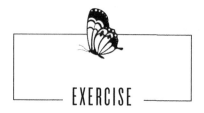

EXERCISE

All exercises are available in the resources pdf:

Mindset exercise

The first exercise is in the workbook pdf and is about your mindsets. This exercise will help you to understand what type of mindset you have and the situations that a fixed mindset can create.

Go through the list of mindsets and identify which of yours are most prevalent. Follow the link to the workbook where you can see some common mindsets, both fixed and growth. Circle which ones apply to you.

Fears exercise

This is a simple journaling exercise that I would like to introduce you to.

Get a piece of paper (space is also available in your workbook) and write down what your fears are. Then write down your desires. Removing anxiety and depression is about moving from your fears, facing them, and aligning your life with your desires. This is not easy to do, but just writing this down on paper is the first step.

Lifestyle change exercise

Eliminating anxiety and depression is also about establishing healthy habits in alignment with your desires, facing your fears and pushing through your mindset. Go to the workbook and, if you want help with working through these, please do contact me to book a few sessions. We can do this together! Check out my blog on **asking for help** (link available in the resources).

SUMMARY

In this chapter we have covered:

✓ Knowing what your mindset is for recovery

✓ Understanding your fears

✓ Taking action or getting help

✓ Improving your general mental health.

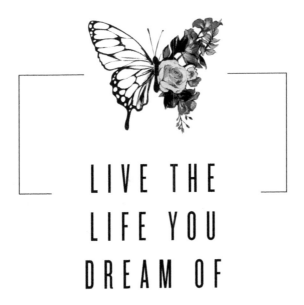

LIVE THE LIFE YOU DREAM OF

"To laugh is to risk appearing a fool
To cry is to risk appearing sentimental and soft
To reach out to another is to risk involvement
To show up and expose your feelings is to risk
exposing your inherent self
To place your ideas, your dreams, your desires
before people is to risk their loss

To love is to risk you might not be

loved in return

To live is to risk dying

To show strength is to risk showing weakness

To do is to risk failure

The greatest hazard in life is to risk nothing

The person that risks nothing, gets nothing, has

nothing, is nothing

He/she may avoid suffering, pain and sorrow,

but they do not learn

They do not grow, they do not live,

they do not love

They have sold and forfeited

freedom and integrity

They are a slave, chained by safety,

locked away by fear

Because only a person who is willing to risk not

knowing the result

Is FREE."

― WILLIAM ARTHUR WARD

One of my dreams in life was to be able to scuba dive one day. I imagined what it would be like being at the bottom of the sea and swimming with the fish in their environment. This was such a strong desire in me. I have always been such a lover of water, and I spent so much time in the swimming pool as a child. It gave me a sense of freedom and peace of mind. In 2012 I received the opportunity to learn to scuba dive.

It was thrilling and scary. After quite a few lessons in the basics, safety and some shallow scuba trips, I went with a group to dive a shipwreck at depth. I was so scared, but this was one of those 'fulfilling my dreams' moments. As I swam around a shipwreck 30 metres underwater, I felt not only exhilaration but a sense of being at complete peace with myself. As we surfaced from the dive, I had such an overwhelming feeling of achievement. I sobbed happy tears on the way home on the ferry as the sense of pride in myself, gratitude for my life and pure joy swept through my body.

If I had not done any of the work on myself in the previous steps of this model, I would not have been able to fulfil this dream. I would not have had the courage to take this risk, because my inner critic would have told me I couldn't do it, and I also would have felt I did not deserve to spend the money on myself for this experience. I would not have asked for help, because I would not have felt worthy. I would not have understood the workings of my brain and my potential to feel anxiety, so I would not have had the tools to manage my anxiety.

My anxiety levels were high throughout the experience, but I consistently self-talked and rationalised my thoughts. My mind was reacting; as my instructor put it, I was in a hostile environment and my survival instincts were kicking in to tell me to get the hell out of there!

WHAT'S THIS STEP ALL ABOUT?

This step is about living the life of your dreams. I will take you through setting goals, taking things one step at a time, not putting pressure on yourself but taking risks in life.

This step is last because it provides a bigger picture; it instils hope of a better future and belief in yourself. It helps you see that anything is possible, and it is the ultimate rebellion against the place you were in at the beginning of your journey. You truly are a rebel once you get to this step.

This step means you can be the person you are truly meant to be, and you will take the action to achieve that. This step may not be easy, but with all the tools you have learnt and implemented in the previous steps, you will be able to achieve it.

You only have one life. Why not live it as best you possibly can? You have achieved so much in your life, and you can continue to do so. You have been carefree and happy before, and you can be again. This step gives you permission to enjoy your life. It will leave you at the end of your life able to look back and say, 'Yes, I lived my life to its best despite the difficult circumstances I was in.' You will have a sense of pride and be free of regret, resentment and self-blame.

WHY IS THIS IMPORTANT FOR YOU?

It is important for you because you have always been a person who has driven for the best in your life, and you are doing it again. Your life has taken a massive turn in direction, but you are fully equipped to face this change now.

The cost of not sorting this out is that you will end up with unfulfilled dreams and ambitions, leading to disappointment but perhaps also a feeling that you are not leaving the legacy you would like. You may continue to feel stuck in that thought of 'What is the point of my life?'

You may also continue to blame others for how you are feeling, which in itself will impact your relationships negatively, bringing sadness, anger, resentment and loneliness to you and perhaps to others. You will continue to feel that you cannot trust other people, as you will not have taken the opportunity to challenge that belief you have developed, and also you will perhaps continue to believe that you cannot trust yourself. I know that, deep down, you know this is not true.

SUSAN'S STORY

When Susan came to me, she told me she was struggling with feeling extremely low and depressed. She said that she kept coming back to this place of intense depression, being tearful, unmotivated and unable to get out of bed, time and time again. She felt so rubbish within herself – lethargic and so, so tired. She said she was spending days in bed avoiding the world, feeling hopeless and just crying all the time.

Susan joined a retreat. She was really quiet at first and was reluctant to speak, but over time, with the other three ladies she was with, she started to share a little bit about how she was feeling.

Susan and I sat down to have a chat together during this time, and we realised there was a pattern to her feeling the way she did. Susan cried a lot in this session. I felt emotional too, being with her, but it was so wonderful to see the hope come back into her eyes that perhaps there was some possibility of changing things. She spoke about her situation at work, which was really affecting how she felt about herself. She worked in a male-dominated environment and felt she had no power there and was treated as the underdog. Susan was so talented and such a wonderful leader, but she did not believe in herself. I really wanted to help her find that belief and peace of mind as she so deserved this.

The pattern she felt she was stuck in was that she would get a new job and feel extremely excited about it, work hard and put everything into it. This would include staying late at the office, working weekends, and then drinking for her time out and relaxation. She was also 'eating on the run' too often, not picking healthier options for her body and mind. If a project ended or the pace of work changed, if there was uncertainty in her employment or if she received a knock-back, she would feel deflated. This would start a slide in her mood. Eventually, she would slip into feelings of depression, which could last for weeks. Susan told me that she would then just look for another job, thinking that was what she needed to resolve how she was feeling. She would get another job... but then find herself back in the same situation a year or 18 months later. Susan was feeling so frustrated with her life; she said she felt like a failure and consistently told herself she was not good enough.

Susan and I worked together intensely on her inner critic. We explored books together, completed exercises about that voice in her head and identified when the inner critic was taking over. Susan started to be able to 'talk back' to her inner critic and, as her confidence built, she started to believe that it was actually OK for her to be who she was. This was massive for her.

Part of the 'educating about the brain' stage for Susan also involved educating her about her feelings. Susan was not someone to recognise how she was feeling, so this often would get pushed to the side, resulting in her overworking at times. We worked on this using feelings diaries and always using the language of 'How are you feeling?' I think Susan got fed up with me continuously asking this question, but it was so key for her being able to take control of her mind and body. Susan brought in routines, with my help, of mindfulness, meditation, yoga, exercise, good food, rest and lots of great self-care.

We explored what she really wanted in life – not what she thought she 'should be' but who she really is. She built a collage of her dream life and then started to take some risks, with my support, implementing her dream life. This involved getting a puppy, a complete relocation to her dream home, a change of job to something less pressurised, and a complete change to the types of holidays and recreational activities she was engaging in. As she started to put all this in place, the depression began to slip away.

Susan built a daily log/journal which addressed all of her self-care needs and goals on a daily basis. She started to really implement these and also put in some boundaries in her working life, to help her stay safe from the burnout she had been experiencing. All of this was put in place with the help of my accountability and support.

Susan's confidence began to build, and she started to become more aware of her thoughts and feelings. She could now take control before her emotions became destructive, taking action and making the changes she needed to get herself back on track.

Moving out of the city into the countryside was a massive step. Changing her lifestyle, focusing on her relationship, getting a dog and reducing the unhelpful behaviours – such as her drinking and unhealthy eating habits – were all part of the process, and she achieved them with my help and support.

The result was that Susan is now really living the life of her dreams. She has a new home in the countryside, away from the pressure of the city, and a less pressured job. She spends more time on what matters to her in life; the things that are important to her and make her happy. Susan is now able to manage her work pressures, so she is not staying late to work or compromising her wellbeing with work commitments.

Susan's pattern had been a two-yearly cycle of emotional breakdowns, so that is why we worked together for so long. The two years passed with no breakdown. In fact, just happiness and getting used to the less pressured life were her main difficulties; there was no overwhelm. I know that sounds contradictory, but she genuinely struggled with the whole concept of feeling happy and not being busy all the time. There were, of course, moments of self-doubt, but Susan was going through a massive transition and transformation to living in accordance with her true self and values. This was something she had never done before. In this process there were a lot of old ideas to let go of, as well as fears. We worked through these together.

Susan started to feel happy on a daily basis, not just because she was achieving at work but because she was connecting with her husband and enjoying time with her dog and being in nature. Susan really felt at peace with her life, and the inherent fear of going back to depression started to ease off. Susan started to feel confident that she knew how to manage slight setbacks and that they did not mean everything was falling apart. She felt sure she now had the tools to pull herself through difficult or challenging times and felt equipped with everything she needed to help her. She was more in tune with her feelings, so was able to pre-empt difficulties and schedule in time and activities that supported her emotional and mental wellbeing. She felt like she had more energy, rather than being tired all the time and running on empty, just waiting for the next holiday. She no longer felt the need to drink alcohol to help her relax after a hard and stressful day; walks with the dog in the countryside and the mindfulness techniques were sufficient to manage her stress.

She also was able to take it a lot easier on herself, so she was not feeling so guilty all the time. The feeling that she was failing started to slip away. Susan was confident that she was doing the best she could and was also sure that her needs were important, even though they might be different from what she had believed they were before. Susan had started to live the life of her dreams in alignment with who she truly was.

HOW TO LIVE THE LIFE OF YOUR DREAMS

Goals

The first thing you need to do in this step is to set your goals. You can do this in a variety of ways – you can get creative or you can just write them down – but it is important to spend some time doing this.

Doing this provides you with a 'bigger picture', a 'vision' of where you want to end up. Having this is powerful in itself, because you have almost imprinted it on your brain.

By having this imprint you will be more inclined to work towards your goals as opportunities or decisions are presented to you. Even though this process is science

"Remember that you can only do this one step at a time; things happen in their own time, and if your goals are not being fulfilled immediately it does not mean you are failing"

based and all about your thinking and conditioning of your brain, it can feel quite magical.

Try to keep a positive mindset about your goals; see them as something you *can* achieve rather than letting thoughts like 'This won't happen for me' or 'I am not deserving of this' creep in. Challenge those fixed mindsets.

Patience

The other thing you need to do is to be patient. Remember that you can only do this one step at a time; things happen in their own time, and if your goals are not being fulfilled immediately it does not mean you are failing. Sometimes things will change quickly and sometimes they will change slowly, but now you have set your goals, things can start to move towards them being fulfilled.

In the introduction to the book, we saw an exercise called the Cups of Life, which is really useful and can support you with this.

The Cups of Life will help you to define how you are feeling about different areas of your life and so decide which areas are a priority to work on. This in turn will help you to become more rounded. We can try to ignore the bits that are not going well, but they will leave an element of negativity. Of course sometimes there are things we cannot change but– with a little thinking outside of the box, some personal reflection and maybe some help– you will be amazed what areas you can change in a positive way.

For instance, if your relationship is going well but you are struggling with your money management, perhaps this would be an important area to focus on.

Do not put pressure on yourself, but be aware of the fact that resistance may come up – so be prepared to get support from others to help you push past your comfort zones. Remember that resistance is only natural. Get some support if you can, whether that is joining a support group or letting a family member or friend know what you are doing and asking them if you can get their support for a while. This will allow you to talk things through with them, discussing and exploring your progress.

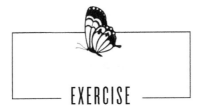

EXERCISE

All exercises below are available in the resources. Follow the QR code to access them.

Complete the Cups of Life

This exercise is in the workbook PDF. Follow the instructions to complete the Cups of Life.

Goal setting

Write a list of your goals after completing the meditation, which is available in the resources.

Or get some paper magazines, pens and glue. Make a collage: cut out pictures and draw on a piece of paper anything related to what comes up for you.

SUMMARY

In this chapter we have covered:

- ✓ How to set goals

- ✓ Why setting goals is important

- ✓ Your approach and mindset to your goals

- ✓ Taking risks, a step at a time

- ✓ Using lists to write down your goals

- ✓ Using collage to write down your goals

- ✓ Using the Cups of Life to see where you are in terms of life's goals.

WHAT NEXT?

While we have come to the end of this book, we are only at the beginning of your journey and your new life.

As we come to the end of this journey together, I just want to say, 'Well done, you!' You have done so much by getting to the end of this book and now you have the toolkit to get you started on your journey towards having peace of mind.

If you have completed some of the exercises, I offer even bigger congratulations. Are you feeling the effect of doing the work? I expect so. I am so proud of you. You really have taken the first step towards feeling better and being happier within yourself. In fact, you have done the hard bit just by making a commitment to something as a starting point. Now you need only continue finding support and information to help you get to the 'life of your dreams', back on track, with the misery behind you and great coping strategies to help you through the rest of your life.

You are now able to feel more positive, understanding yourself more and feeling less out of control. You can even put yourself first now! Wow, what an achievement. Do not minimise the brilliance of this, as it is not easy to do. Well done!

However, this is just the beginning. Imagine how you would feel in a few months' time if you continued this journey, using these methods to go a little deeper and understand yourself a little better, learning more tools for positivity and peace of mind along the way. Life could be so different for you. So what are you going to do to keep moving forward?

You have so many possibilities open to you now.

A simple next step would be to become a part of the Crystal Clear Retreats Community – you could visit us on Instagram as @crystalclearcoach or Facebook as Crystalclearretreats. That would be a wonderful way to ask any questions or to start to meet like-minded people.

Remember: we are stronger together. Whoever they are, finding 'accountability buddies' can be a huge help along your way. You can do the gratitude challenge together or compare notes on your Cups of Life or your goal collages. It's always so much easier and more fulfilling doing this with someone else. After all, you can share experiences with each other and learn from each other.

Amongst the book's resources you can access the *free* video series on the '7 Pillars to Overcoming Depression' or go to **www.crystalclearcoaching.org** to help you to keep putting one foot in front of the other on this journey. You could go further, in fact, and access one of my REBEL method workshops (also available on the resources page – follow the code below with your phone's camera).

If you use the code 'book 22' you can have a 10% discount on our prices. Beyond that, you could really take a leap and join one of my retreats. Book a call with me now to have a personal chat about what we can offer, or send me an email at:

vanessa@crystalclearcoaching.org

I would love to meet you somewhere along the way, whether that is in person or online, whether it is in passing or as a guide.

I wish you all the best now, and I have a warm feeling writing this knowing that you have come this far by rebelling just a little against the life that has been limiting you and that you have seen some of the benefits you can gain from it. I am with you in heart and mind and, if you have any doubts or concerns that might stop you from making the progress you need, please feel free to contact the community.

Do let me know if you have read this book and send me a review. I would love to hear your thoughts.

Take care and remember **you are worth it.**

I believe in you!

Printed in Great Britain
by Amazon